Fit & Healthy Pregnant

MOM IN BALANCE

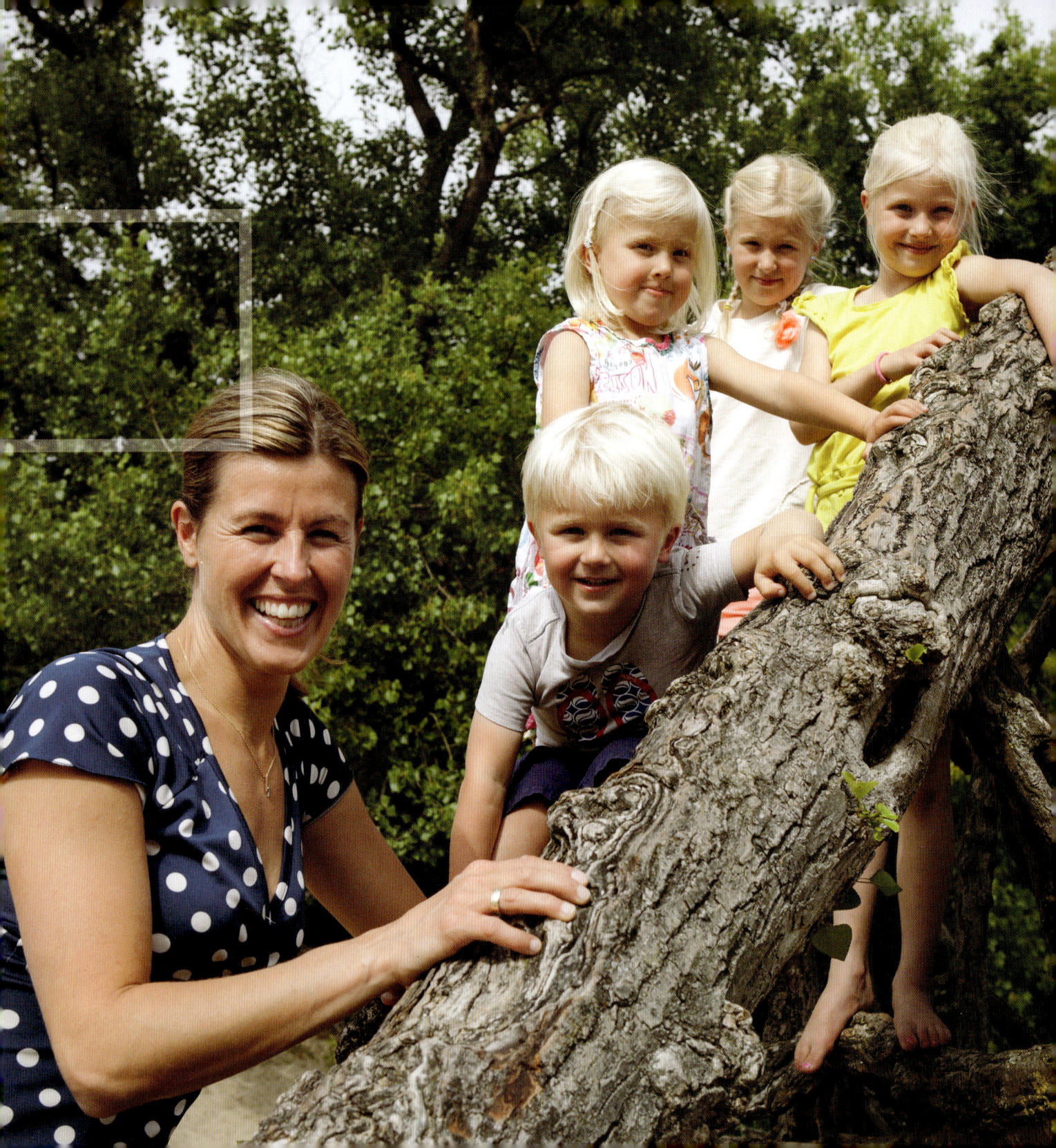

About Mom in Balance

As a mother of 4 wonderful children I have experienced how exercise and healthy nutrition have a significant impact on your pregnancy and recovery after giving birth. In our workouts I see on a daily basis how sports and exercise influence the way women experience their pregnancy in a fit and healthy state and are able to keep a high energy level during the first years of motherhood.

The first years with your children are genuinely considered hard work for which you do need all additional energy available. By already living healthy and active during your pregnancy you will notice you have more energy during the first years of family life. This way you will be able to deal much better with all other demanding aspects in your life.

Outdoor activities are my passion

For several years I have cycled and ice-skated at a considerable high level in Holland, an experience I could put to use to train other people. I have studied for and worked as a medical nurse plus studied at the Vrije Universiteit in Amsterdam for organisation-anthropologist. Before we moved to New York in 2005 I worked as a Health Care manager for a team of home-care nurses. At New York University I studied for Life Coach and attended a personal training course at the American College of Sports Medicine.

New York

Early 2005 I gave birth to our first daughter and when she was 9 months we moved to New York. During our stay there it was remarkable to see how many women remain active during their pregnancy. It was not an exception to see 8 month pregnant women running their laps in Central Park. Seeing this was my major inspiration to start Mom in Balance!

Pregnant with our second daughter I started to give training and coaching to pregnant women and mothers in Central Park in New York City. After having done so for 2 years we moved back to Amsterdam and my experiences in the United States formed the foundation for Mom in Balance in The Netherlands.

With this book I really want to inspire and assist you to experience a fit and energetic pregnancy. Using my own knowledge and experience as a basis and with the input of experts in the area of pregnancy, gynaecology, sports and nutrition I have composed this workout program.

Gynaecologist Dr. Petra Bakker provided the medical input for an active and healthy pregnancy. Pelvic physical therapist Heleen van Kuyk advised on the strengthening of the pelvic floor muscles. Nutrional expert and dietician Lillian Hentzen shared her knowledge on the area of nutrition during pregnancy. Lillian owns a dietician practice specialised in this field.

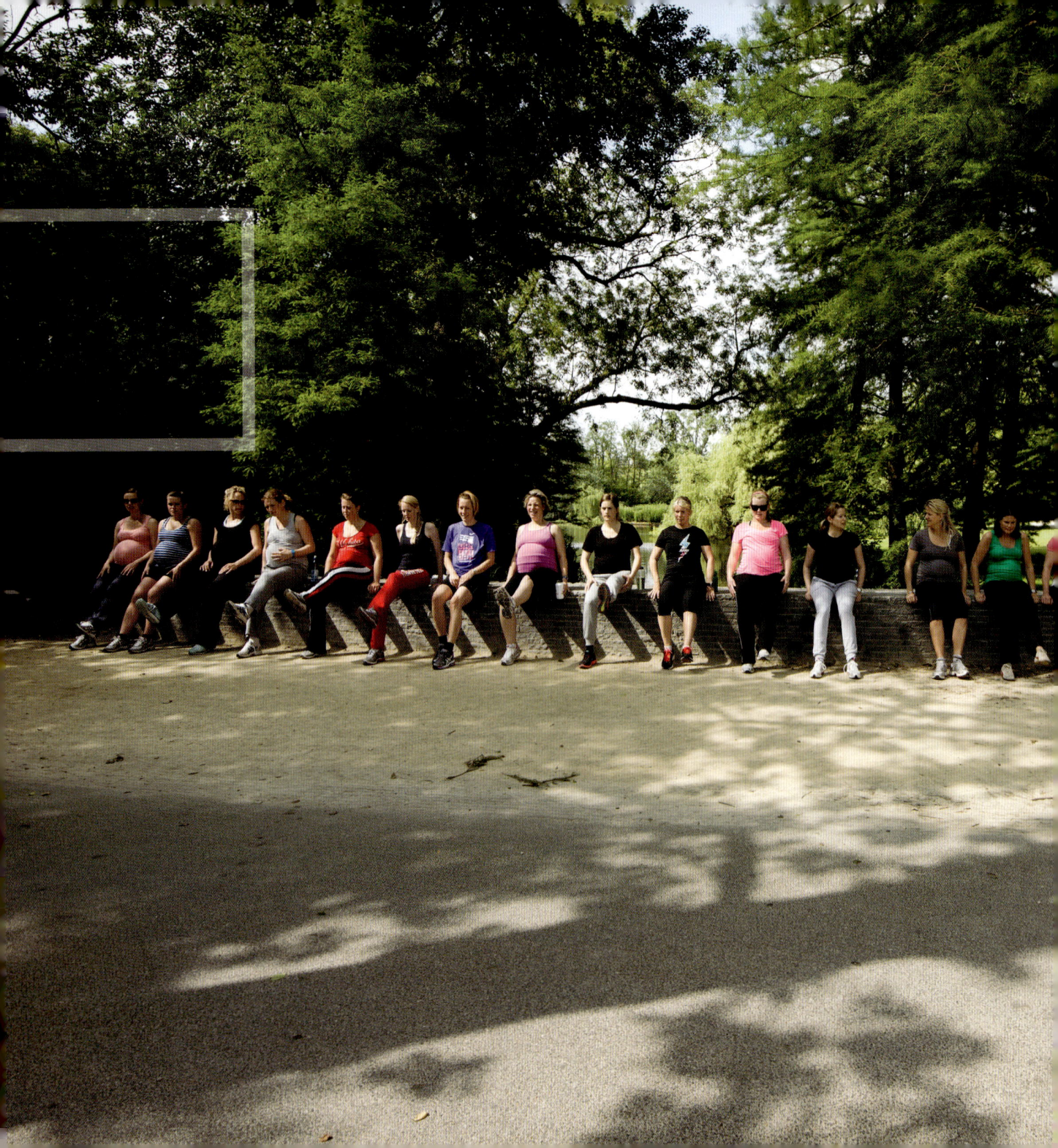

What this book can mean for you

This book provides you with a workout program directed to each of the 3 trimesters of your pregnancy. With this as your guide, you can stay active in a responsible way in each trimester. The Mom in Balance workouts consist of various cardio, muscle enhancing and stretch exercises. For each trimester I will indicate which changes your body will be going through and how you can adapt your workouts to those changes.

The Mom in Balance workout program advises trained women who want to continue their exercises and also women who want to start sports while pregnant. So if you have not been able to do any sports the last few years this is an excellent time to start. You do however have to take it slowly at first. During our Mom in Balance training courses, mostly the same questions arise:

- Is exercise safe for the baby?
- Until which stage can I train my abdominal muscles?
- Which sports can I continue doing and which really can't?
- Can I continue exercising all the way to the end?
- Can I still run/jog during my pregnancy?

This book provides an answer to all these questions.

When reading this book it will mean you'll have to get into action too!! I will hand tips and tricks on how to carry on your exercises during the full period of your pregnancy. All the advantages of exercise during pregnancy will be discussed, after which you will make your personal action plan. In the 9 month fit journal which you will find in the back of the book you can keep record of your sport activities. This should serve as a stimulus to keep a regular schedule of workouts and exercises.

In the journal you can also write down the physical changes that you notice during the 9 months. Make pictures of your belly each trimester and put the photos in the frames, this way the book becomes a great record of your whole pregnancy!

Use Fit and Healthy Pregnant the coming nine months to optimally enjoy your pregnancy and feel strong and energetic!

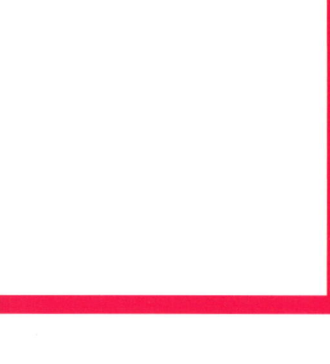

Contents

About Mom in Balance   5
Contents   9

[Chapter 1]
Stay fit for you and your baby   11
Advantages of sports
and a healthy diet   12
Your pregnancy:
working to a healthy balance   16
Action plan   17

[Chapter 2]
Exercise and pregnant   19
Basic guidelines   20
Cardio-fitness   22
Stretching and strong muscles   24
Pregnant: which sports can you do   25
Suitable sportswear   27

[Chapter 3]
First trimester   29
Physical changes   30
Hormonal changes   32
Exercise in the first trimester   34
Cardio-fitness   36
Stretching   41
Strong muscles
   - legs and buttocks   44
   - upper body   48
   - abdominals   51

[Chapter 4]
Second trimester   53
Physical changes   54
Exercise in the second trimester   58
Cardio-fitness   61
Stretching   64
Strong muscles
   - legs and buttocks   66
   - arms   68
   - pelvic floor muscles   70
   - abdominals   71

[Chapter 5]
Third trimester   75
Physical changes   76
Exercise in the third trimester   79
Cardio-fitness   80
Flexible muscles   84
Strong muscles
   - legs and buttocks   86
   - upper body   88
Exercises to relax   91

[Chapter 6]
Healthy nutrition   93
Nutrients   94
Vitamins and minerals   99

[Chapter 7]
Recovery after delivery   103
First six weeks after birth   104
Your changing body   107
Exercise post birth   111
Cardio-fitness   113
Getting stronger   115
Flexible muscles   118

Finally   121

Journal   123

Colophon   162
Index   167

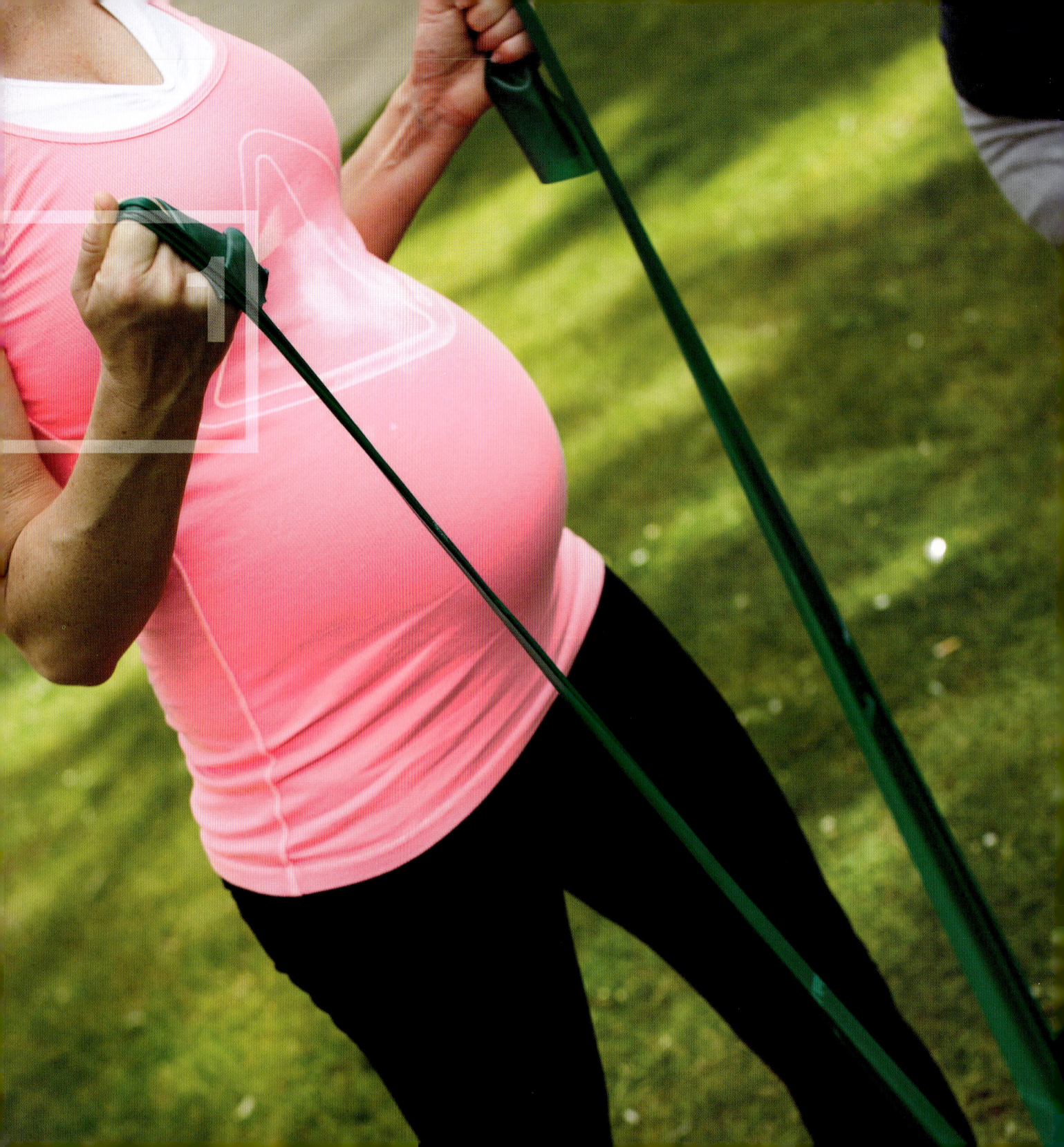

Stay fit for you
and your baby

Great, you're pregnant!

The coming nine months your body will be all about growing a healthy baby! This will demand energy, focus, discipline, perseverance and a strong body. Being pregnant is top-league sports for which you can definitely use extra energy. Exercise and healthy nutrition can make a huge difference in how you feel the coming months.

This first chapter will inspire and stimulate you to exercise, eat healthy and to keep on doing so during the full 9 months. First I will explain the advantages of sports and a healthy diet. More and more research is being done into the impact of exercise during pregnancy, the results of which will be discussed here.

In the second part of this chapter you will put together an action plan for your fit and healthy pregnancy.

Advantages of sports and a healthy diet

1

[Chapter 1]
Stay fit for you and your baby

Various studies show that exercising during the pregnancy offers clearly demonstrable advantages. The American gynaecologist and expert on fitness during pregnancy Dr. James Clapp and the Canadian doctor Michelle Mottola have by far done the most elaborate research in the field of sports during pregnancy. Already from the 70s on they have been studying the effects of exercise during pregnancy on mother and child. I will discuss here the positive effects that sports and nutrition offer during your pregnancy.

Improved condition
Staying active will keep your condition at the pre-pregnancy level the coming nine months and it may even improve. Exercise on a regular basis increases the maximum amount of energy a woman can generate and the amount of oxygen she can use per minute (Clapp, 2002). Research shows that even a maximum push is well possible during pregnancy. When pregnant physical strain does not have to mean any risk for mother or child as long as it is a normal pregnancy without any complications (Paisley, 2003).

Van Doorn (2009) too indicates that there is no evidence to assume intensive exercise increases the chance to a miscarriage or premature birth.

Less pregnancy troubles
Research conducted by Clapp shows that regular strength and cardio training prevents many pregnancy ailments or in any case reduces the chance. Tiredness in the first trimester is one of those symptoms you counter by getting into action.

Healthy increase in weight
Continuous exercise and a healthy diet will help you realise a moderate weight increase. Regular workouts enable that stored fats will be used as a source of energy. In the Netherlands currently women are not weighed anymore at their visit

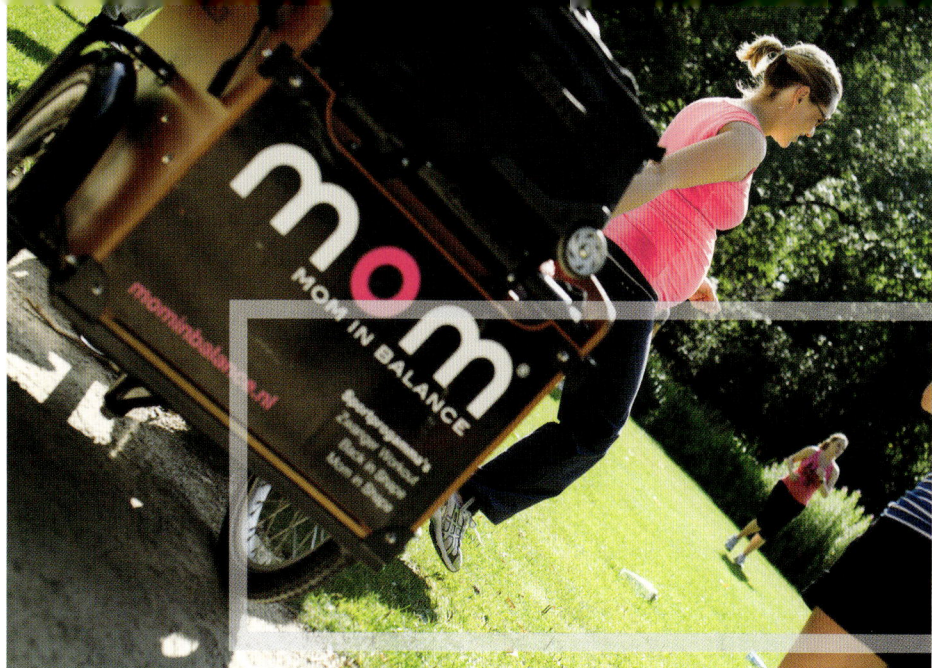

at the obstetrician or gynaecologist. If that is the same in your situation, that weight check will have to be done by yourself. Even if you reach a stage where you do not want to come anywhere near a scale, my advise is to still keep weighing yourself. Keep a record in the journal in the back of this book, this will stimulate to keep a normal weight increase.

One of Dr. Clapp's studies shows that women who exercise regularly gain on average 4 kilos less than pregnant women who have not been active during pregnancy.

A healthy growth of the placenta

Exercising during pregnancy on a regular basis gives a better growth of the placenta (Clapp, Rizk, 1992). When a woman exercises all the way to the end of the pregnancy, the placenta grows on average 3x as fast during the second trimester and will have around 15% more surface, which provides for an optimal living climate for your baby. This will also enable your placenta to function optimally all the way to the end.

The delivery

Continuing your exercises will help you in your preparation for the delivery. Several studies show that a fit and healthy woman has a better chance on a short delivery with less complications and less exhaustion. When you go into labour with a fit body the pain will not be less necessarily, but it will give you a better endurance to have a good delivery (Mikeska, 2004). We get this feedback very often as well from the women who have trained with Mom in Balance throughout their pregnancy.

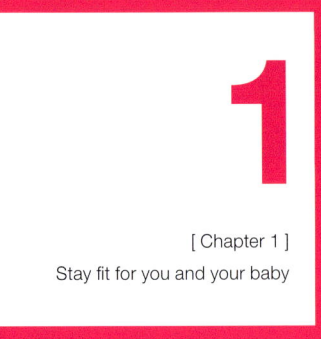

[Chapter 1]
Stay fit for you and your baby

Good for the baby
The healthy environment that the mother creates in the womb by staying active during pregnancy has a positive effect on the development of the baby according to Mottola (2010). She indicates for instance that the chance of chronic illnesses diminishes for the future adult (Mottola et al. 2010). Furthermore, studies done by Richard Nisbett, professor at the University of Michigan, show that doing sports have a positive effect on the IQ of the baby. Children of whom the mother exercised half an hour per day scored on average 8 points higher in IQ tests than children whose mother did not exercise at all (Nisbett, 2009).

A large British study shows that women that continue their exercises during their pregnancy usually get active and sporty children. Which is not so strange according to the researchers as women who are active during their pregnancy continue to be so after their delivery. And especially during the first years children are very susceptible to their parents' behaviour, they often copy their behaviour including the habit of exercises (BCC).

Strong muscles and flexibility
Making your muscles stronger by strength- and resistance training will increase and maintain your muscle power and endurance. This will enable you to move easier during the day. Strong muscles also prevent pelvic and lower back problems in many cases. Regular stretching will increase your flexibility. By strengthening your muscles and keeping them flexible your fitness level will increase and you will feel fit throughout the whole pregnancy (Bosch, 2007).

Sleep better
Many pregnant women have more trouble sleeping during their pregnancy, which makes them feel more tired during the day. By putting your body at work with a workout routine you will notice you will fall asleep more easily. You will also sleep deeper as your body is recovering from the activities. This deeper sleep results in more energy during the day.

A good mood
Sports and healthy food creates a better mood. After your workouts you will feel very satisfied because of the endorphins which are released during sports. Endorphins are natural substances created by the body during physical activities. You will be rewarded immediately after your workout with an energetic and happy feeling, and you will be very relaxed after the workout.

Balance
An active and healthy lifestyle will support you in combining your pregnancy with your job, family life and all other things that are important to you. Because you want everything else in your life to go on as usual of course.

After the delivery
Last but not least, also the recovery after labour and delivery will be much easier when you did your exercises and enjoyed a healthy diet. You will notice you will fit into your pre-pregnancy clothes much faster.

10 REASONS TO STAY ACTIVE DURING YOUR PREGNANCY

1. You feel fit and healthy and will have more energy
2. It has a positive impact on your child
3. It keeps your condition up or it even improves
4. It contributes to a healthy increase in weight
5. You will have less pregnancy ailments
6. You will sleep better
7. Your endurance will be better before, during and after your delivery.
8. Bouncing back faster to your pre-pregnancy shape.
9. It is relaxing and keeps you in a good mood
10. Doing sports with other pregnant women is stimulating and you meet new people

Your pregnancy: working to a healthy balance

1

[Chapter 1]
Stay fit for you and your baby

Get into action right away! When you manage to stay active already at the beginning of your pregnancy, you will immediately feel the tremendous benefits. If you're not sure yet whether exercising during the first three months is safe for the baby, let me reassure you. During the first trimester you can keep on doing all the sports you already did before you got pregnant. Doing sports during the first months of your pregnancy does not entail any extra risks (Clapp, 2002)

Feeling more tired and/or sick during the first trimester usually means you need some extra motivation to remain active. Sometimes you are already glad you got through the day. But especially now it is important you get into action. By exercising you will feel much better. And this time you not only do it for yourself, but for your baby too!

How do you find the motivation, time and energy to maintain a sports routine?

Top-league athletes perform best when they have a clear and motivating plan. As you are about to perform at top-level yourself these 9 months, write down an action plan! This motivates and stimulates to keep moving.

Stay fit, energized and balanced

Action plan

Make your own action plan now, by following the next three steps

Step 1 Brainstorm
Do some brainstorming. Take a piece of paper and write down everything that comes to mind when you think about your health. The Mom in Balance Wheel of Life can be an inspiration here. In this model you will find all the important aspects in the life of a mom-to-be.

Step 2 Write down your goals
Take a look at the things you wrote down. What are the two most important reasons for you to feel fit and energetic during your pregnancy? For instance, if you wish to keep on working full-time as long as possible, do you want to work out to keep your body in shape, or do you want to have enough energy each week to go out with your friends? These are your personal goals which you can achieve with the Mom in Balance sports program. Write down your goals on the page here.

Step 3 Your own action plan
With your own goals as the basis to start working out with the Mom In Balance sports program, write down your action points regarding your exercise and diet plans. These points will help you achieve your goals. Each trimester you will compose a new action plan, using the insights from your bodily changes you have experienced plus the workout advises from this book. This way you can adjust your action plan to your personal situation each trimester. If you wish to start straight away, see page 35 to make your action plan for the first trimester.

Goal 1

Goal 2

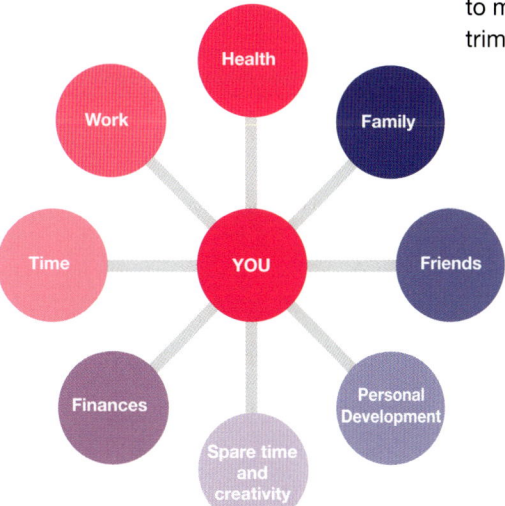

MOM IN BALANCE 17

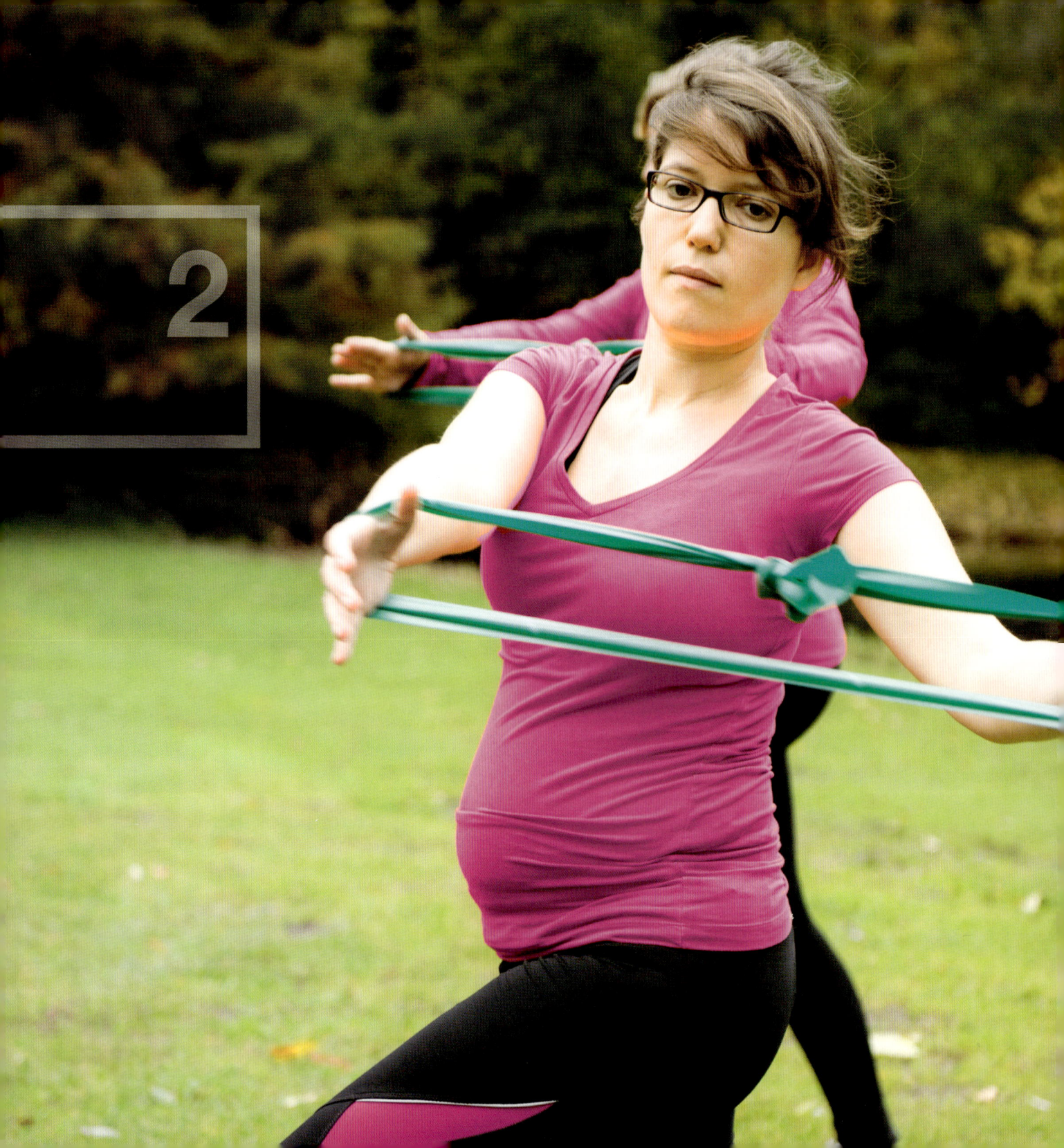

Exercise and pregnant

Stay healthy and energetic!

During a normal pregnancy you should be able to continue your exercises until right before going into labour. Your body will undergo considerable changes because of the baby growing inside you, which will make you have to adjust your training schedule. In this chapter I will give you directives on a responsible workout schedule. I will also explain about the types of activities that are most suitable while you are expecting.

Basic Guidelines

2

[Chapter 2]
Exercise and pregnant

Now you are pregnant it is even more important to listen to your body while exercising. To stay active the coming nine months in a healthy and responsible way, I advise you to keep to the following basic guidelines with regard to temperature, intensity, hydration, diet and fatigue. Also, before you start exercising, always consult with your doctor or obstetrician before starting this or any exercise program.

Temperature

During your pregnancy it is important that while exercising your body temperature doesn't run up too high. When you keep up your hydration and if you are fit, you can regulate your body temperature more efficiently and will experience less fluctuations in temperature during your workouts. To keep your body temperature down it also helps to wear clothing that is not too tight and to do your sports in a cool environment, preferably outside. (Artal et al. 2010)

Intensity

As indicated before, various studies show that intensive exercises during pregnancy do not entail more risks. Most studies indicate that your maximum heartbeat should stay between 130 and 145 heartbeats per minute (Mottola et al., 2010). You can check the intensity also quite well by the talking test. As long as you can still talk during training, you are doing fine. When you run out of breath you reach the limit and the point your muscles start to get acidified. This happens when you do your exercises with a high heartbeat and keep on exercising until your muscles feel sore. The lactic acid produced as a waste by your body causes the acidification of your muscles. Acidified muscles can influence your hormone balance. That is why I advise you to exercise up to a maximum of 70% of your capacity during pregnancy, to prevent acidification. At the beginning of your workout you could feel this sooner so do make sure you build up your training slowly. When your muscles get trained more and more or when you already are well trained at the start of your pregnancy, acidification will not happen that fast.

Lots of fluids, eat well, more energy

Hydration

Make sure you drink a lot during your workouts. The increased blood volume causes a higher need for fluids. Next to the recommended 1.5 litres, I advise you to drink at least 2 glasses of water more per day than what you drank before you got pregnant. So make sure you always carry water or a sports drink with you during exercising. A good indication is 1 glass of water every 20 minutes you are active.

Nutrition

While expecting your metabolism increases and you burn sugars faster. During your workouts you need carbohydrates, as they provide fast energy. Make sure you always had something to eat before your exercises and you take a snack rich in carbohydrates after sports. For more advice on nutrition check chapter 6.

Fatigue

Because the development and growth of your baby totally depends on your body you get tired more easily during your training. Do not wear yourself out entirely. On some days when you already have been quite active you might not have the energy to do your workouts. Do not do one then, just take a nice 20 minute walk or bike ride or you even might just need a nap to get new energy!

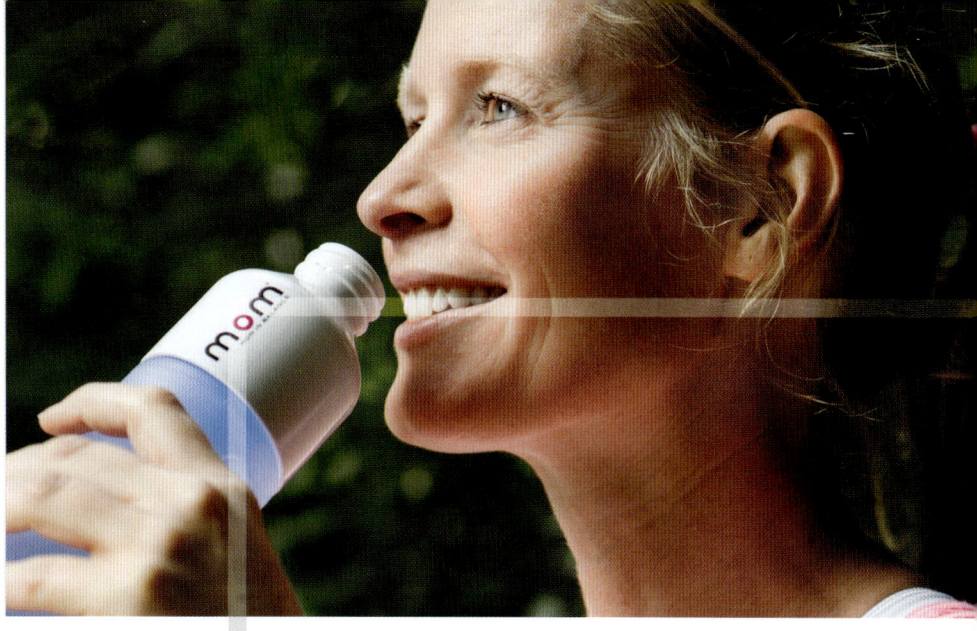

Basic guidelines summed up

1 Make sure your body temperature doesn't increase too much
2 Train at max 70% of your capacity, and your heart rate shouldn't exceed 145 beats per minute
3 Drink plenty of water during your workout
4 Take a carbo rich snack before and after exercising
5 Do not wear yourself out completely
6 Don't exceed 1 hour of sports per workout

On top of these basic guidelines there are always the regular rules: do a 5 minute warm up before your workout for a good blood circulation. This way you prevent all sorts of injuries. Stretch at least 5 minutes after your training.

Stretching exercises can be found in chapters 3, 4 and 5.

Keep up your hydration during your workout

MOM IN BALANCE

Cardio-fitness

2

[Chapter 2]
Exercise and pregnant

Cardio-fitness increases your endurance. The condition of your heart and lungs improves and you are definitely going to need that during your pregnancy and delivery. A strong heart better provides your hardworking muscles with fresh blood, which enables your muscles to get into action at the right moment. The more energy and stamina you have the coming nine months - and especially during the moment supreme- the better!

Cardio-fitness is a heartbeat-increasing exercise. Your body produces endorphins, which make you feel good. And it is relaxing too.

It is important to know how you can become fit or stay fit during pregnancy. But what is the best way to train your heart for the big delivery 'challenge'?

What do you gain from cardio-fitness during pregnancy?
1 More energy
2 Good condition of your heart and lungs
3 Endurance
4 A relaxed and happy feeling

Walking
Going for a walk is great for everyone who is planning to start exercises. After all, it is the easiest way to get into action. You do not need any special clothing, just a pair of good (walking) shoes, light clothing and off you go.

Jogging
If you already were an enthusiastic jogger before your pregnancy, you can easily continue doing so during while expecting. As long as you feel fine, you can keep on jogging (recreationally) until far into your pregnancy. If your growing belly and breasts eventually start to become uncomfortable, you can go for a bike ride, a walk or a swim instead. Use the jogging schedule on page 39 to keep your condition up.

Tips for walking and jogging
A good posture is of course always important, but definitely when you wish to change your walk into a workout. When going for a walk and/or jog, make sure to keep the following in mind:
- Keep your upper body straight. This will create less pressure on the pelvis during your walk.
- Keep your arms relaxed in a 90 degree angle alongside your upper body. Make sure your hands do not

CARDIO-FITNESS

There are three cardio sports you can do best during pregnancy: going for a walk or jogging, swimming and cycling.

pass the body and your elbows not in front of the body.
- Remind to breathe well during your walk
- Relax your belly and pelvic floor as much as possible during the walk
- Wear a good, supporting bra
- Good walking shoes are important
- Stay hydrated, bring along water or a sports drink

Swimming

Assuming you can swim reasonably well, this is the best moment to go to the swimming pool. After all, in the water you weigh about 90% less than outside the water, which could be a relief. When swimming you strengthen your muscles without burdening your joints, which especially now is a big advantage. For a sound swimming workout your swimming posture is important. Professional instructions during your pregnancy are therefore advisable.

Tips for swimming The following basic rules for swimming will help you make your swimming workout during pregnancy safe and effective:
- Quietly breathe in and out. Take a good breath of air every two strokes.
- Try to make long strokes. You should aim for less than 25 strokes per 25 meters.
- Stop swimming if your pelvis starts to bother you. When breast stroke feels uncomfortable, try to swim slower and keep your legs closer together, or change to another stroke.
- Find out more about special pregnancy-swimming courses in the vicinity.

Cycling

You can still ride a bike during pregnancy, outside on a flat road as well as on a home trainer. Cycling can also be fitted in easily, by for instance going to work by bike instead of the car. If you ride your bike regularly, you will work to keep a solid condition. Also, cycling does not burden your joints.

Tips for cycling This way your bike ride stays pleasant and you prevent injuries:
- Start your bike ride slowly, as a warming-up
- If you have a bike with gears, try to cycle as light as possible.
- Sit up straight on your bike
- Make sure the height of your saddle has been adjusted to your body.

Cross-training

Cross-training is actually quite simple. It means you combine several kinds of exercise. This gives a bit of diversity and is a great training. By doing different kinds of sports you use different muscles every time. The variation can also help you stay motivated to keep on exercising.

The cardio-program means you have to plan a 30 minute cardio-workout at least 2 times a week. You can go for a walk, ride your bike, go spinning or swimming. Make sure you do not plan the same activity twice in a row and also fit in at least one day of rest. Next to the cardio-workouts use the exercises in this book for a total body workout. After your workout please allow 5 minutes to stretch.

Or ... a combination of all three!

MOM IN BALANCE

Stretching and strong muscles

2

[Chapter 2]
Exercise and pregnant

Stretching
Stretching is good for many reasons: it prevents your muscles becoming stiff, your body will be more flexible, and it improves your blood circulation, which reduces the risk of injuries. Your body will become stronger, it relaxes your muscles and gives an energetic feeling. In short: stretching is a good addition to your cardio-workout and exercises to strengthen your muscles. You will find stretching exercises in chapters 3, 4 and 5, specifically suited for each trimester of your pregnancy.

What do you gain from stretching?
1 Supple muscles and joints
2 Relaxation
3 Energy
4 Prevention of injuries

Strong muscles
Muscle strengthening exercises will make your body stronger. Your coordination and posture will improve and you will feel more flexible. Next to that your condition improves and it prevents excessive weight gain. It also helps you stand up straight when you become heavier on the front side. Your body will stay in top shape! In chapters 3, 4 and 5 you will find muscle strengthening exercises, specified for each trimester.

What do you gain from muscle exercises?
1 Strong muscles
2 Powerful feeling
3 Energy
4 Good posture
5 Coordination and flexibility

Pregnant: which sports can you do

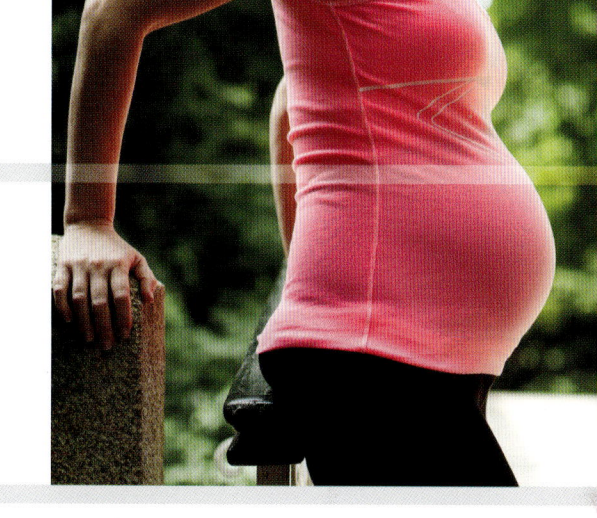

The best sports you can continue doing during your pregnancy are walking, jogging, swimming, cycling and the exercises in this book. If you wish to keep on doing your regular sport, it is advisable to use the following tips.

Your joints will become more flexible when you're expecting, so you can get injured more easily, try to avoid turning movements or sudden stops. Also do your exercises on a flat surface.

From the 16th week you better avoid doing exercises where you can get hit by something in your belly or may bump into other people or where you can fall. For instance tennis, volleyball, hockey and skating. We found that lots of injuries occur practicing these sports.

Skiing is no problem at the beginning of your pregnancy when you are a skilled skier and ski on slopes that are not too steep. Later on during your pregnancy the risk of falling on your belly gets bigger, so I advise you to only take small hills.

Mountain climbing and abseiling are not a problem early in your pregnancy, up to 2500 metres. Above 2500m the air becomes too thin so the baby may not get enough oxygen.

If your belly starts to become bigger, you shouldn't do this sport anymore as the risk of heavily bumping your belly into the mountainside will become too big.

Diving and skydiving are sports you can't do for a while anymore during your pregnancy, as you will be very sensitive to decompression disease.

When do I have to stop doing sports?
When you experience the following symptoms, you should temporarily stop doing any sports.
- High blood pressure
- Dizzyness
- Sudden headache
- Nausea and/or vomiting
- Reoccurring hard stomach
- Vaginal blood loss

Attention!
Always consult your doctor or obstetrician before you start a sports program.

MOM IN BALANCE

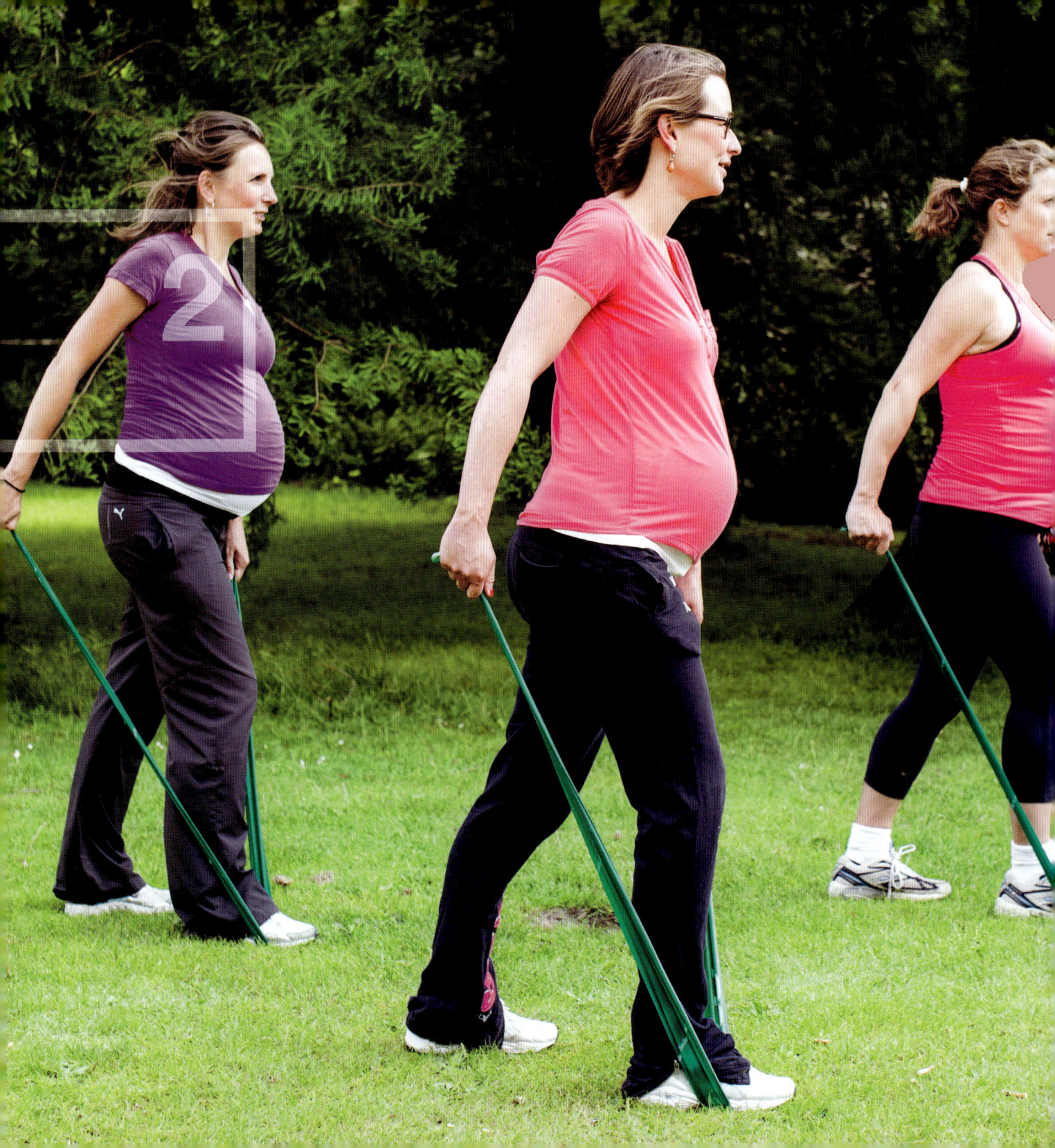

Suitable sportswear

When you workout, you want to be as comfortable as possible. Comfortable sportswear can make a huge difference. Before you start I would like to give you some advice on good sportswear.

Clothing
Sportswear designed specifically for pregnant women is usually made of easy jogging fabric. If you exercise outside I recommend wearing breathable synthetic sportswear. Unfortunately there is not much synthetic pregnancy sportswear available, but one size bigger from the normal collection will do for quite a while. When it's cold it's better to wear several layers of thin sportswear instead of just one item.

Swimwear
There are special swimsuits available for pregnant women, which you can wear until the end. Do make sure your swimsuit is suitable for lap swimming. Choose strong, good quality material as it will give the best support. If your swimsuit has an extra bra/support on the inside that could be quite comfortable too. Goggles are always quite handy, they enable you to keep your eyes open, it is easier to swim your laps.

Sportsbra
As your breasts will grow heavier, it is important you wear a properly fitted sports bra for extra support. Make sure your bra can grow during your pregnancy, go to a lingerie shop for advice. If necessary just wear two sports bras on top of eachother.

Shoes
Preferably, wear supporting and shock absorbing sneakers during sports. Wearing proper shoes helps to avoid your joints to get overstressed, therefore reducing the risk of injuries.

Maternity support belt
Nearing the end of your pregnancy it can be very comfortable to wear a support belt for extra support of your belly, back and pelvis. You also relieve your womb ligaments, especially when your belly is quite big. When you still actively jog and exercise, it's important to make sure your belly gets extra support. It also relieves the lower back.

Where can I find the right sportswear?
Suitable sportswear can be found in sport shops. Get advice from an expert when you want to buy the right sneakers. Via the Mom in Balance web shop we offer as many products as possible to make exercising during pregnancy as comfortable as possible.

For more tips and clothing, check:
www.mominbalance.com

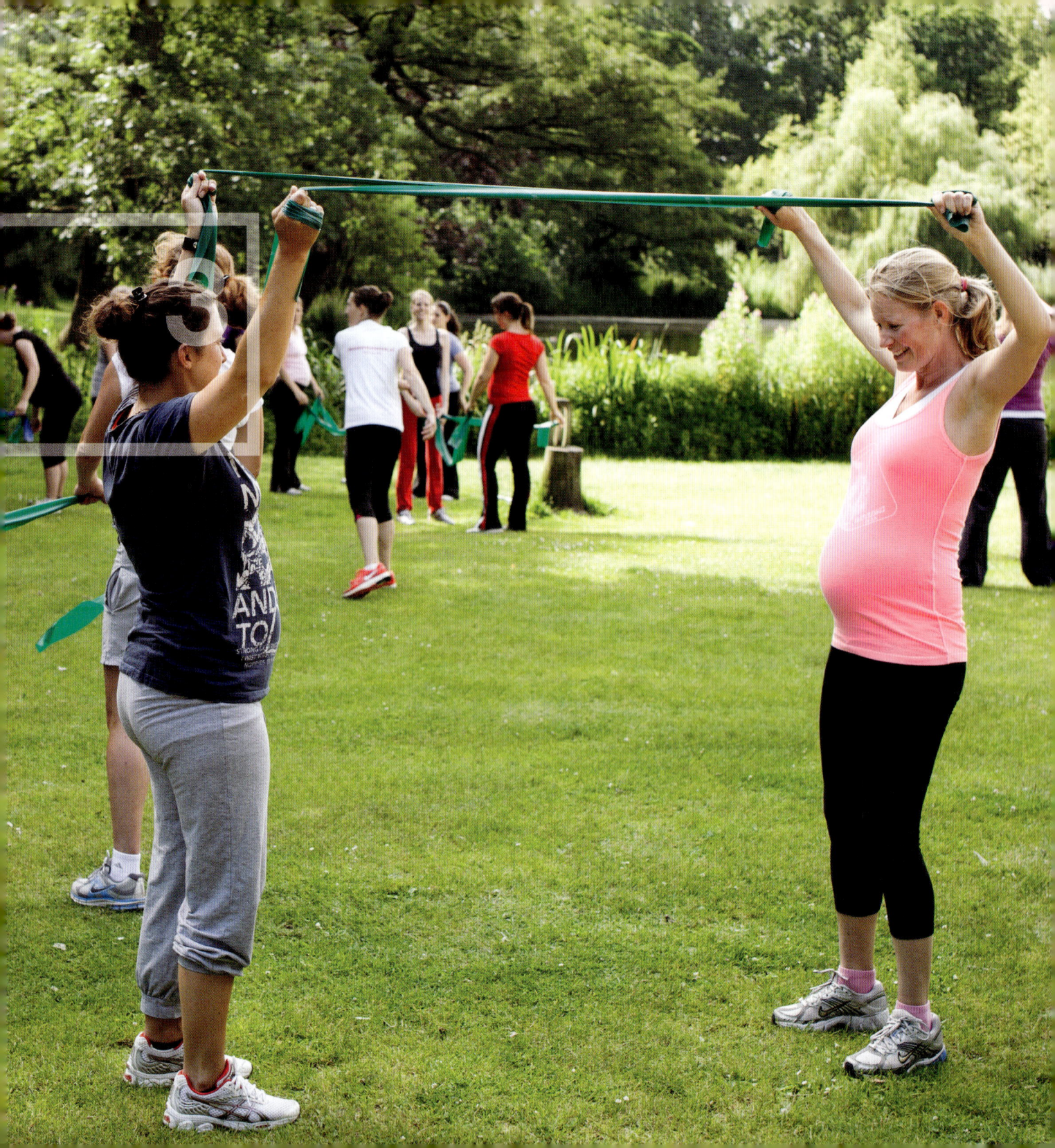

[1] First trimester

Week 1 to 13

The first trimester of your pregnancy runs from week 1 to 13. Now that you know for sure that you are pregnant and slowly get used to the idea, you probably experienced the first symptoms already. You know that your belly will grow much bigger, but will also discover that being pregnant means your whole body is changing. Feeling more tired, sick or more emotional because of all those hormones running through your body may be quite upsetting. And exercising may not be the first thing on your mind. But particularly in the first trimester of your pregnancy you can lay the foundation for a fit and healthy pregnancy!

In this chapter you will discover which physiological and hormonal changes will occur during the first trimester. When you know about these changes, you can adjust your sports program to it. That way you will be active in a safe and effective way.

Physical changes

[Chapter 3]
First trimester

During the first trimester your whole body will be prepared to build a healthy home for your baby. Probably lots of bodily changes will occur. These are the most important ones:

Increase in blood volume

During your pregnancy you will need to pump blood for two (or more). This means your body needs to produce more blood. At the end of your pregnancy your blood volume may have increased to up to 2 litres more than normal. Your circulation system is expanding so fast, your heart needs to work extra hard to keep up. So it is quite logical your heart beat is higher than before your pregnancy.

Your body is working hard, so you may get tired sooner during your workout or you may feel a bit lightheaded. When you feel dizzy during your exercises, take it a bit slower and lower the intensity of your workout.

Weight increase

During the second month of your pregnancy your scales may already indicate you've gained weight. How much you will gain each trimester is different for every woman, so it may be you didn't gain anything during the first months - because you were feeling sick e.g. - but you will catch up again during the months you feel better. On average you gain about 12 kg during your pregnancy. Nowadays many women gain more than the average increase in weight. By staying active and eating healthy it will be easier to keep those extra kilos around the average.

After the delivery you lose about 5 kg and during the first few weeks after that another 4 kg. The kilos that remain are fat reserves for the period you will breastfeed, on average about 2 kg, but also that varies for each woman.

Bigger breasts

During your pregnancy the weight and shape of your breasts change. Your breast volume increases because of the following three changes:
- Increased blood circulation in the first trimester
- Increased number of lactiferous ducts
- Increase in size of lobules, especially during the last 8 weeks.

These changes are normal. They may however, have some consequences for the sports you still find pleasant to do. A proper sports bra is essential. Make sure you wear the right bra all the time and have your cup size measured, allowing some space for extra growth during your pregnancy.

Frequent bathroom visits

The pregnancy hormones, growing womb and increased blood circulation of your kidneys work on your bladder. That is why you may have the feeling that, especially during the first months and last few weeks of your pregnancy, you have to go to the ladies room more often. And even though it may not always be very practical, it is normal, so do not try to compensate by drinking less. During sports you need to keep up your fluids, so do drink enough.

WHERE DO THE EXTRA KILOS COME FROM

Baby	3,5 kilo
Womb	1,0 kilo
Placenta	0,5 kilo
Extra blood	1,5 kilo
Breasts	0,5 kilo
Extra fat reserve	3,0 kilo
Extra fluid	2,0 kilo
Total	12,0 kilo

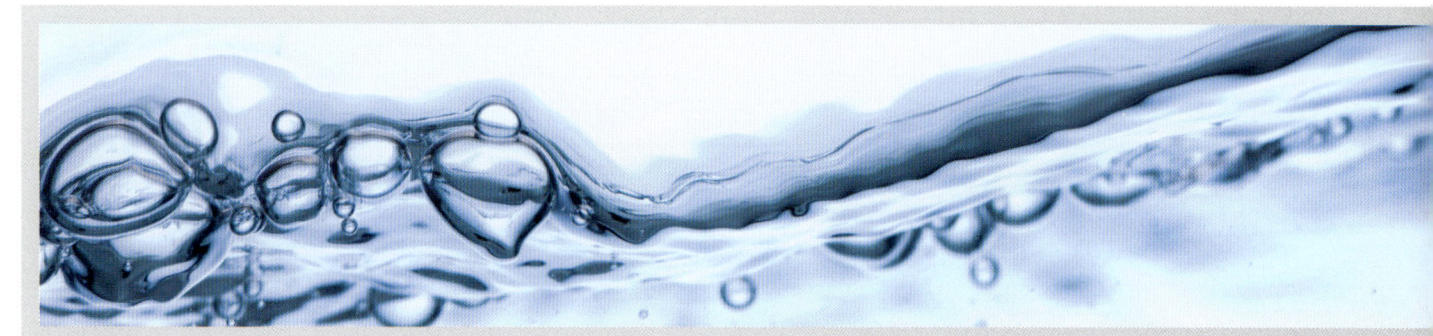

MOM IN BALANCE

Hormonal changes

[Chapter 3]
First trimester

Pregnancy hormones immediately go to work and let your body know that a baby is on its way. Next to the fact that those hormones may cause mood swings and may give you a feeling your brain is not working properly, they have another function. They make sure that at the beginning of your pregnancy your whole body is getting ready for the baby. Thanks to those hormones the placenta starts growing to create an optimal environment for your baby.

The three most important hormones that get to work during your pregnancy are:
- Progesterone
- Relaxine
- Oestrogen

Progesterone
Immediately from the first week of your pregnancy your body produces the progesterone hormone. Progesterone makes your joints loosen a bit and makes sure your womb can grow without contracting. Next to that the progesterone causes you to be out of breath sooner during physical strain. This is because during your pregnancy your body has to work harder to get rid of the CO_2. This is how it works: progesterone makes your breathing centre (in your brains) more sensitive to CO_2. This increases your incentive to breathe and gives you an increasing feeling of shortness of breath. So do not think your condition suddenly went down to zero, because this all is part of the game. And don't let yourself be shocked - you can continue your workouts just fine.

Progesterone - Relaxine - Oestrogen

Relaxine
Relaxine is probably the most important hormone to take into account during exercising. This hormone is produced already early in the pregnancy - after the second week- and stays active until about 4 to 6 months after the delivery. It mainly makes your joints more relaxed and supple. It mainly makes your joints more relaxed and flexible, which helps your body carry the baby and eases the delivery.

Next to the pelvis, other joints also become more flexible. This increases the risk of injuries, so do listen to your body. Make sure you walk or jog on a flat surface, to avoid spraining your ankle.

Oestrogen
Oestrogen is also a very important hormone active during a pregnancy. It is responsible for the growth of your uterus. During your pregnancy your uterus increases in volume, up to 5 litres!

Oestrogen also prepares your breasts for lactation. The normal weight increase is realized by oestrogen. Furthermore it takes care of the distribution of extra fat that you will store in various places in your body during your pregnancy.

MOM IN BALANCE

Exercise during the first trimester

3

[Chapter 3]
First trimester

Exercising during the first trimester of your pregnancy may be confusing. Although you may have developed a bigger belly and your breasts feel like milk is going to be produced right now, you cannot show that you are pregnant yet. During the first trimester it Is fine to continue doing any sports you already did before you became pregnant. The baby will not be hurt as it is swimming around safely, well protected by the amniotic fluid.

Try to keep on doing your workouts right from the start of your pregnancy. It will help you get through the first three months much easier. First write down your action plan to motivate yourself to start your pregnancy as active and healthy as possible. Here you have some tips to carry out your action plan successfully.

Tip 1: Do not aim too high and make a realistic plan. E.g. take a 15-minute walk 3 times a week, even if you wouldn't have mind walking for half an hour each day. This way you will succeed sooner in your plan, and all the extras are just nice.

Tip 2: Mix and vary with different activities. Do a bushwalk instead of your weekly walk in the neighbourhood, and go to your work on your bike. Try to plan two different activities each week.

Tip3: Reward yourself, it really works. Reward yourself at the end of the week when your plan has worked. Go to the movies, or enjoy a lovely facial or massage. This will make sure you will be totally motivated again at the start of the next week.

WORKOUTS DO HELP!

"This pregnancy is quite different from the first one. Despite the fatigue I felt energetic and fit, sporting really does help. With my first pregnancy I immediately stopped exercising, I felt quite unsure and thought it was better to rest. Now, with professional support, I notice I can do much more than I thought and I feel strong en I feel good. With a 1.5 year old at home I lift quite a lot and strong muscles in the lower back, belly and arms are a big help!'

Marianne, Mom in Balance participant

Write down your action plan

Write down your action plan here for the first trimester. Mention how often you would like to exercise and how you intend to start eating healthy. For instance, 'Monday I am going to train with the Mom in Balance Pregnancy Workout and on Thursday I will go walking and Saturday morning I will start working on the exercises', and/or 'Each morning I start with a shake of fresh fruit'.

Action 1	
Action 2	
Action 3	

Tip 4: Don't wear yourself out. If it is one of those weeks you just get nothing done, relax. You are pregnant, so it is quite alright to indulge in this feeling once in a while and do absolutely nothing.

Tip 5: Each form of exercise is good, You really do not have to workout in the gym for hours, it is more important that you find something you really enjoy. If you do the exercises from this book twice a week for 20 minutes, you are already well on your way.

Tip 6: Do sports together. Find a workout buddy or participate in the Mom in Balance Pregnancy Workout for even more incentive and nice contacts with other exercising pregnant women.

Tip 7: An energetic evening. Especially when you are still working 5 days a week, or when you finally have your kids in bed by 8 and your house tidy, it is for many a challenge to get off the couch. Go and sit on the couch with a book or in front of the TV and relax for a while, but do not lie down yet. Do not relax for more than 15 minutes and then get up again. Do your exercises, or go for a short walk and you will notice you will get a boost.

Tip 8: Record your sporting moments in your journal. This way you will not forget a workout that fast and you are less inclined to cancel your workout. The diary motivates and stimulates you to start working on your action plan and it makes you feel good when you keep it up.

Cardio-fitness

3

[Chapter 3]
First trimester

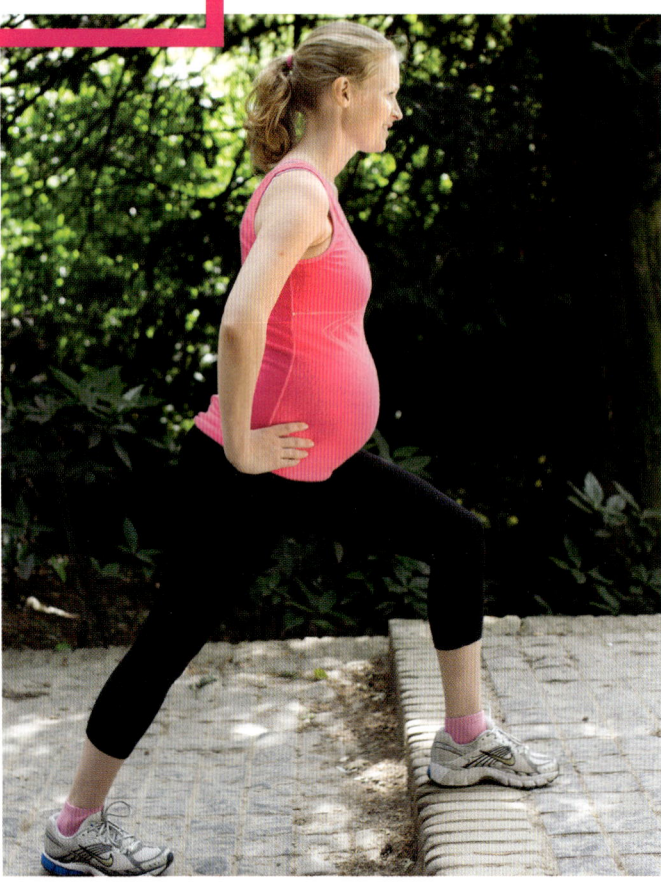

Great that you use your pregnancy as a reason to start exercising! Your body may not be used to regular activity, so you have to build it up slowly. You may ask yourself how much and what you can handle. Will putting on sportswear and motivating yourself take more energy and time than exercising itself? Will you be completely out of breath already at the end of the street? Well, if you keep to the schedules below, you will be fine!

The first thing you have to remember is that your muscles do not have to hurt after a workout. Pushing yourself beyond the point it feels comfortable is bad advice to everyone who is exercising, but it may even be dangerous if you are pregnant. You don't have to walk for hours, every 5 minutes you can squeeze in is already a good start.

CARDIO-FITNESS

Use the different cardio schedules for the beginning and trained athlete.

Are you ready! - beginning athlete

Below here I will mention the sports that are perfect to start with. With this walking program you can make your walks effective and build it up slowly to a workout of 30 minutes max.

Walking

Walking is the best and easiest method to gently start your activities. You can do it wherever you want and it gives an enormous boost of energy. You can make your walk very effective and expand it to 30 minute walks with this walking schedule.

Walking schedule

Warming up: walk for 5 minutes at a slow pace. Then another 5 minutes a bit faster. You must still be able to keep on talking. Always end your walk with a cooling down of 5 minutes, during which you keep on walking at an easy pace. Walk these 15 minute sessions at least 3 times a week. Keep on doing this during the first 3 to 6 weeks. Then expand your schedule by increasing the fast pace by 5 minutes until you reach 30 minutes, warming up and cooling down included.

Swimming

Swimming is a very suitable sport to start with during your pregnancy. Find a swimming pool in the neighbourhood and use the swimming schedule below to build up slowly.

Swimming schedule

To warm up, always start with 5 to 10 minutes in an easy swimming tempo, 2 - 4 laps of 25 meters. For the first three sessions:

Swim 2 laps, rest for 1 minute
Swim 4 laps, rest for 1-3 minutes
Swim 2 laps, rest for 1 minute
Swim 4 laps, rest for 1-3 minutes
Swim 2 laps in a slow tempo

This workout, during which you swim 16-18 laps, will take about 20 minutes. If you think it is easy, you may increase the distance, but do this slowly to keep the motivation high and not wear yourself out in one session.

For the next three sessions:

Swim 2 laps, rest 1 minute
Swim 3 laps, rest 1-3 minutes
Swim 4 laps, rest 1-3 minutes
Swim 4 laps, rest 1-3 minutes
Swim 3 laps, rest 1-3 minutes
Swim 2 laps in a slow tempo

This workout, during which you swim 20-22 laps (including the warming up) takes about 25 minutes. If you feel good, you can increase each workout with 1 lap extra until you swim actively for 30 minutes max.

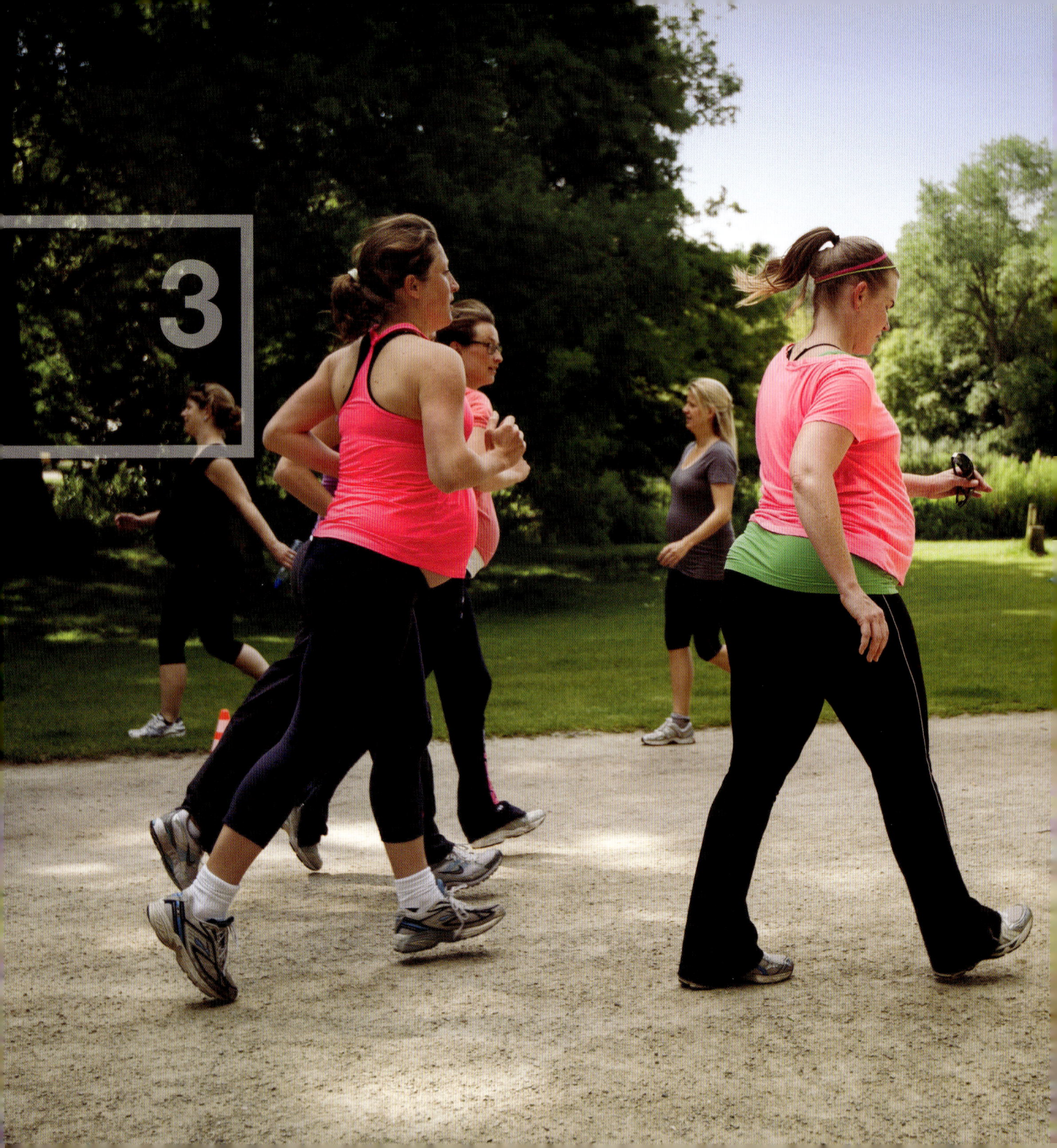

Are you ready! - trained athlete

To start your pregnancy feeling fit has enormous advantages. You are physically strong, you know what your body can and cannot handle, you probably have more energy than women who do not exercise and you already built up a sports routine. Now the biggest challenge probably is trying to keep up your sports routine during the ups-and-downs of your pregnancy.

Because you are used to exercising, you know what it feels like to do sports fanatically -and to get out of breath; and to exercise in a relaxed way, during which you can still talk easily. I recommend you choose the relaxed variation for now. If you normally walk 5 km in 30 minutes, you now will walk only 3 km. Don't feel frustrated. If you keep on exercising with this intensity, your muscle strength and condition will remain at a solid level the coming nine months, and after the delivery you will bounce back better.

Jogging or walking
When you are accustomed to jogging, just keep doing so as long as it still feels ok. It will not bother your baby. Because you will get out of breath sooner now, you will probably not reach the same running speed as before the pregnancy, but don't let yourself be discouraged as you have read before this is just normal physical adjustment.

Jogging schedule
Always start with a 5 minute walk to warm up your muscles. When it does not feel comfortable anymore, slowly reduce the number of minutes you jog and go for a walk instead of jogging.

Week 5-8 Jog for 12 minutes, walk fast for 3 minutes, jog for 12 minutes, walk fast for 3 minutes and end with a 5 minute walk.

Week 9-13 Jog for 10 minutes, walk fast for 5 minutes, jog for 10 minutes, walk fast for 5 minutes and end with a 5 minute walk.

Swimming
Swimming is an ideal sport to do during your pregnancy. It has nearly all the advantages of jogging. Because you continuously push the water away, you strengthen all your muscles. If you wish to compare it with jogging: 1 km swimming equals about 4 km jogging. So if you do 8 km within an hour, you could also swim 2 km. You will use about the same amount of energy and calories.

Swimming schedule
To warm up, you always start with a slow swim for 5-10 minutes, 2-4 laps of 25 meters.

Swim 4 laps, rest 1-2 minutes
Swim 6 laps, using a board, rest 1-3 minutes
Swim 8 laps, rest 1-3 minutes
Swim 6 laps using a board, rest 1-3 minutes
Swim 2 laps in a slow tempo.

This workout, during which you swim 28-30 laps, will take about 25-30 minutes. Total workout of 28 laps = 700 m.

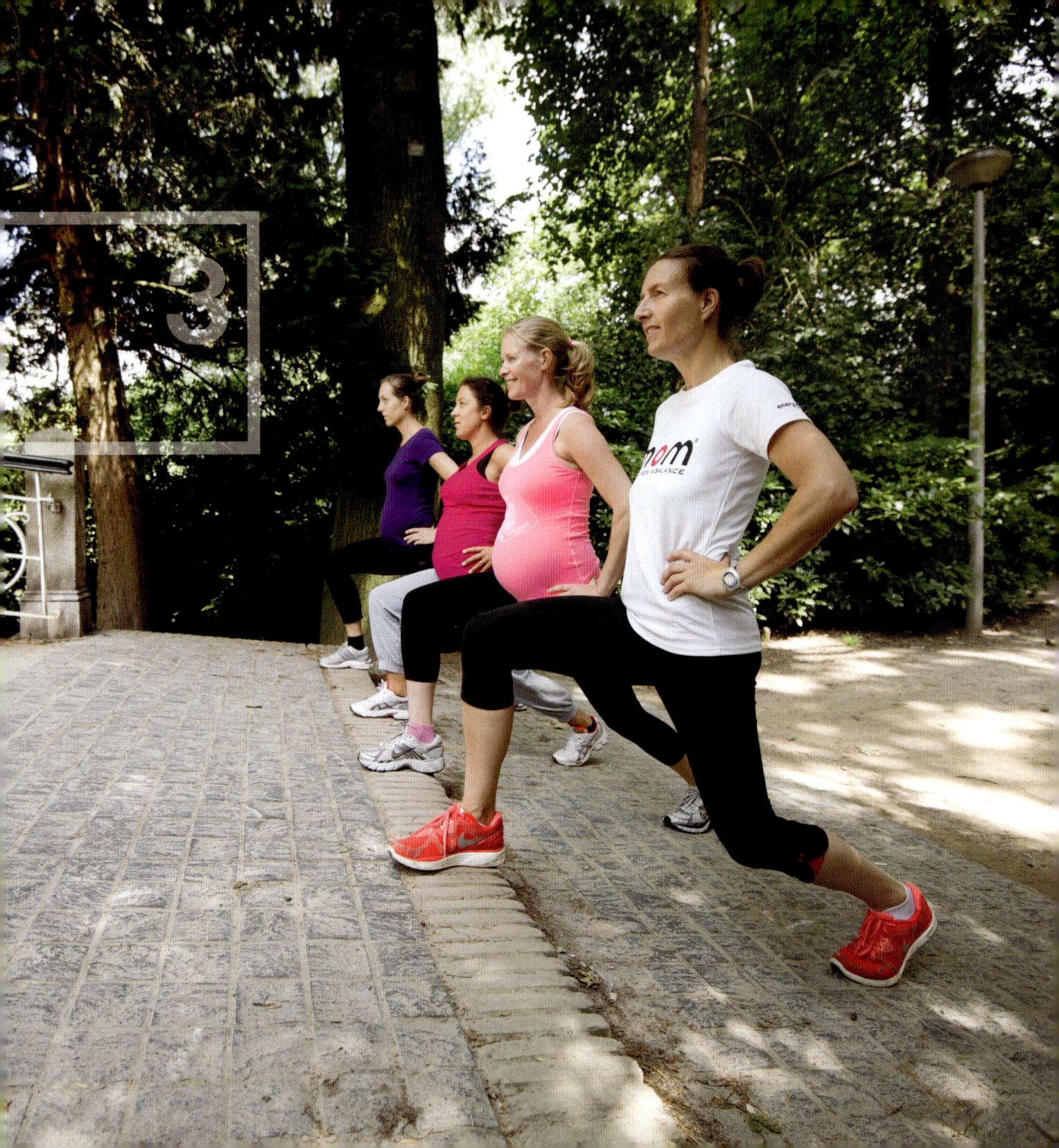

3

Stretching

Always make sure your muscles are warm before you start your stretching exercises. As already indicated before, the relaxine hormone causes your joints to be more instable. That is why you have to be extra careful when you stretch and make sure you do not overstretch your muscles. Try to end your workout with a stretching session as well, as it helps the recovery of the muscles and prevents injuries. Below you will find various stretching exercises for the upper- and lower body you can start with during the first trimester.

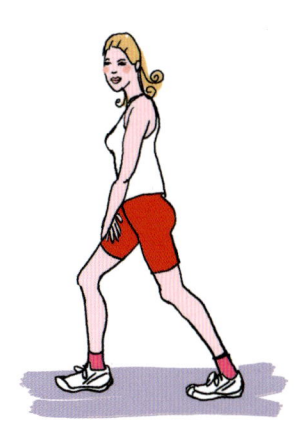

Calf stretch

With this exercise you stretch your calf muscles, and improve the blood circulation of your calf. This can be very useful when you suffer from a fit of calf cramp!

1 Take a big step backwards with your left leg and bend your right leg. Move your weight to your right leg.
2 Keep your left leg straight and press your heel into the ground.

Hold this stretch for 10 seconds and repeat with your other leg.

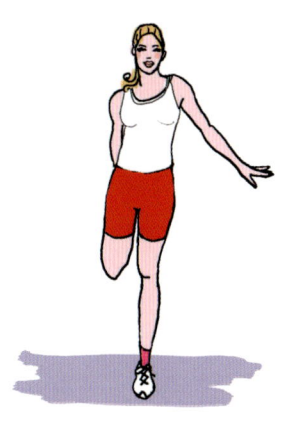

Upper leg stretch

If necessary, hold on to a chair for support when you stretch your upper leg muscles.

1 Stand up straight, keep your knees together and bring your right foot towards your buttocks.
2 Take your right ankle with your right hand and bring the heel to your backside. You can feel the stretch on the front of your upper leg.

Hold the stretch for 10 seconds and repeat with the other leg.

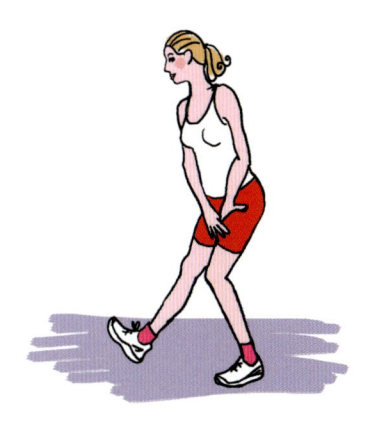

Hamstring stretch

Hamstrings are the muscles that run alongside the back of your thighs to your bum.

1 Take a step forward with your right leg and keep it stretched in front of you with your heel on the ground. Keep your left foot flat on the floor.
2 Move your weight to your left leg and bend your knee.
3 You feel the stretch in the hamstring of your right leg.

Hold the stretch for 10 seconds and switch to the other leg.

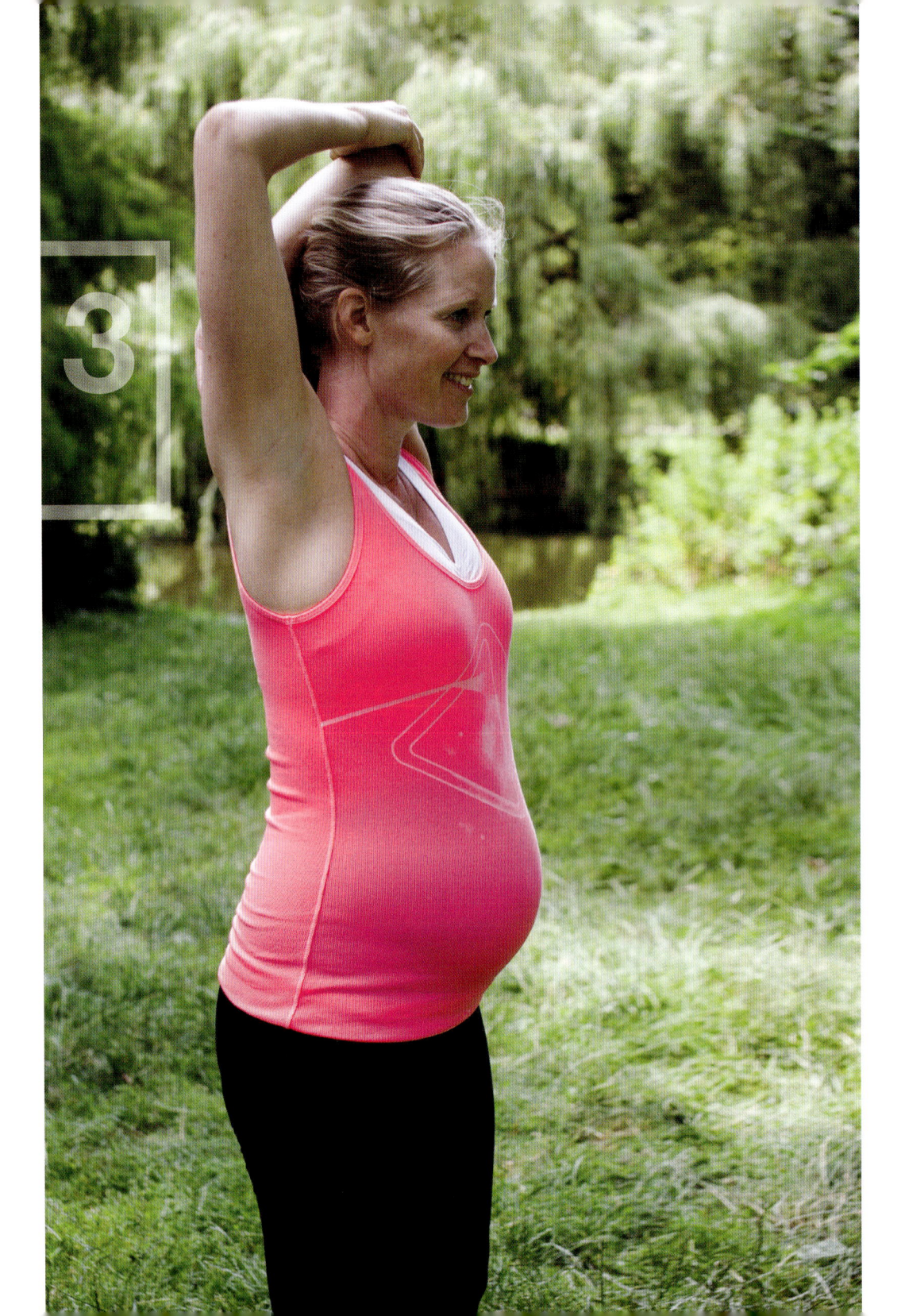

3

Stretching

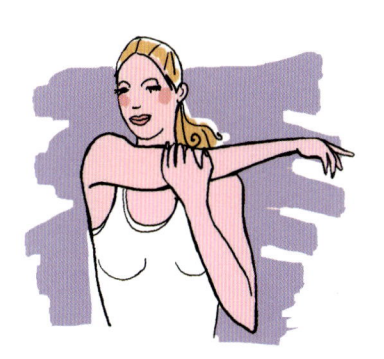

Shoulder stretch

This stretch will make your shoulders flexible. It also helps remove any tension.

1. You can do this stretch either sitting or standing up
2. Grab with your left hand the back of your right arm between your elbow and shoulder and pull your right arm slowly in front of your chest. The stretch can be felt on the inside of your right arm and alongside your right shoulder-blade.

Hold the stretch for 10 seconds and change arms.

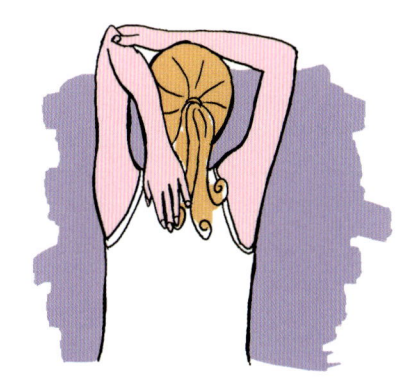

Triceps stretch

You find the triceps on the back of your upper arm. Stretching the triceps is very good for the blood circulation.

1. Stand up with your feet under your hips and your knees slightly bent.
2. Lift your left arm above your head and bend your elbow so that your hand lies in your neck.
3. Take your left elbow with your right hand and pull your arm lightly to the right. This makes your left hand go down automatically further between your shoulder blades. Keep your chin well up to avoid tension in your neck.

Hold the stretch for 10 seconds and change arms.

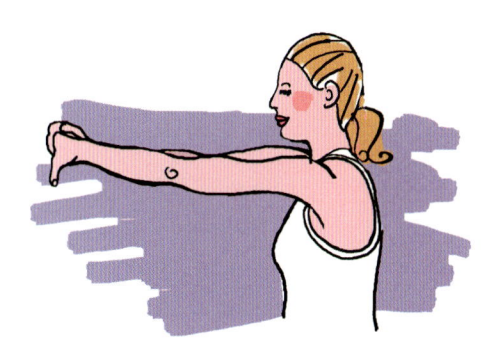

Upper back stretch

Stretching the muscles in your back helps to keep them flexible. If you feel tense or stressed, your back is the first place where muscles tighten.

1. Stand up with your feet under your hips and your knees slightly bent.
2. Intertwine your fingers and turn the palms of your hands forward, then stretch your arms forward as far as possible.
3. Relax your upper back by lowering your shoulders into a relaxing position.

Hold the stretch for 10 seconds.

Flexible muscles - relax - energy

Strong muscles - legs and buttocks

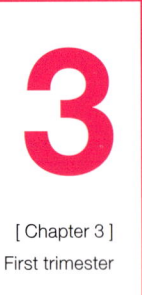

3

[Chapter 3]
First trimester

With the following muscle strengthening exercises you can start immediately in the first trimester. For best results I recommend to do all exercises at least twice a week.

When you do the muscle strengthening exercises for the upper body, it is important you stretch your legs and tighten your backside muscles (glutes). This prevents you from getting your strength from your lower back.

Furthermore I recommend to warm up your muscles before starting the workout. Try to plan the exercises after a walk or -if you stay home- start by a 5 minute sturdy walk on the spot.

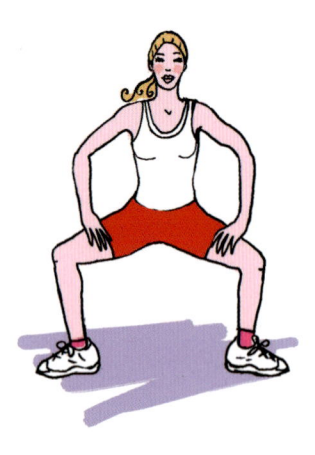

Wide squat

With the wide squat you train your inner thigh muscles. Next to that you train the front and back thigh muscles which is a good preparation for the delivery.

1. Stand up straight with your feet wide. Your feet are turned outwards and you hold your hands on your hips.
2. Tighten your abdominal muscles, push your knees outwards and lower yourself by bending your knees.
3. Lower yourself as much as possible and then push yourself up again from your heels until you stand up straight. Keep your knees slightly bent.

Repeat this exercise 10-12 times.

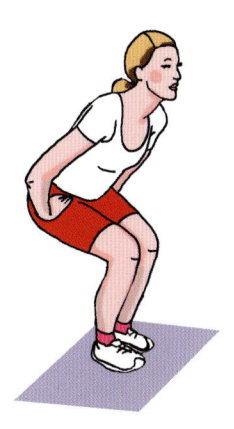

Narrow squat
With the narrow squat you strengthen your butt- and upper leg muscles.

1 Place your feet close together and put your hands on your hips. Do not look at the ground, but face forward.
2 Bend your legs as if you are going to sit down. Make sure you do not topple forward with your upper body and that you only lower your bum. Your knees stay apart.
3 Hold this position for 5 seconds. Then stretch.

Repeat this exercise 6 times. Hold the lower position for another 10 seconds and move slightly up and down.

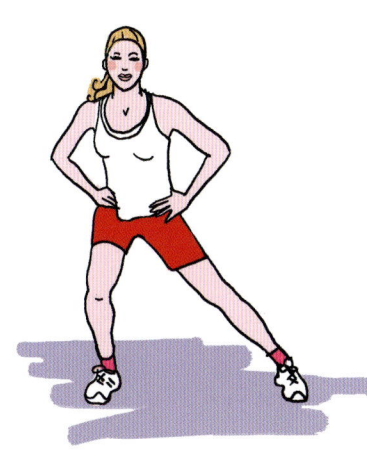

Sideways squat
The sideways squat strengthens your inner thigh muscles and your butt stays nice and firm.

1 Stand with your feet straight at hip-distance apart and put your hands on your hips.
2 Then take one big step sideways and lower your right knee. Move all your weight to the right leg. Do keep both feet firmly on the ground.
3 Push yourself upwards with your right foot and rise to starting position.

Repeat this exercise 6 times to both sides.

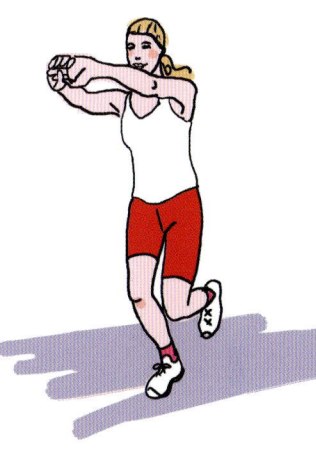

Single knee-bend
This is a good muscle strengthening exercise for butt, thighs and calves. But also a good balancing exercise.

1 Stand up straight and keep your abs tightened. Bend your left leg backwards until it's a 90 degree angle, with your toes pointing backwards.
2 Bend your left knee downwards, bringing your right leg knee straight above your left foot.
3 Stand up straight again.

Repeat these exercises 6 times with both legs.

3

[Chapter 3]
First trimester

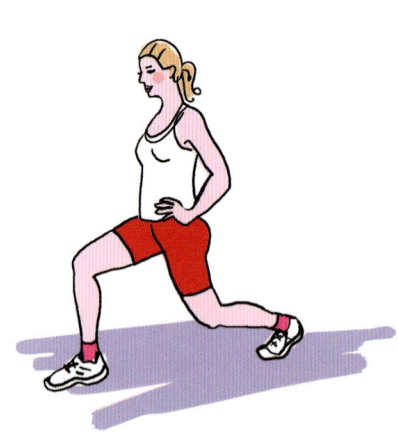

Forward lunge
With this exercise you train your upper legs and glutes.

1. Stand up with your feet spread at hip-distance and put your hands on your hips.
2. Step forward with your right foot and lower your left knee 3 times.
3. Push yourself back up from the right foot to a standing position.

Repeat these exercises 5 times with both legs.

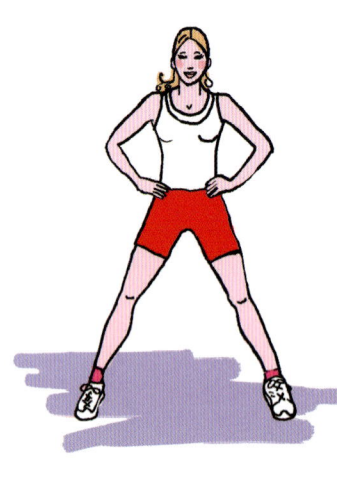

Squat
This is a very effective workout to strengthen the muscles of your legs and buttocks. The squat gives you a stronger lower body, which is very useful in this stage.

1. Stand up with your feet spread under your hips. Keep your arms stretched in front of you.
2. Keep on facing forward and go down with your knees, while pushing your buttocks backwards.
3. Return to a standing position after 5 seconds.

Repeat the exercise 8-10 times.

Strong muscles - upper legs - glutes

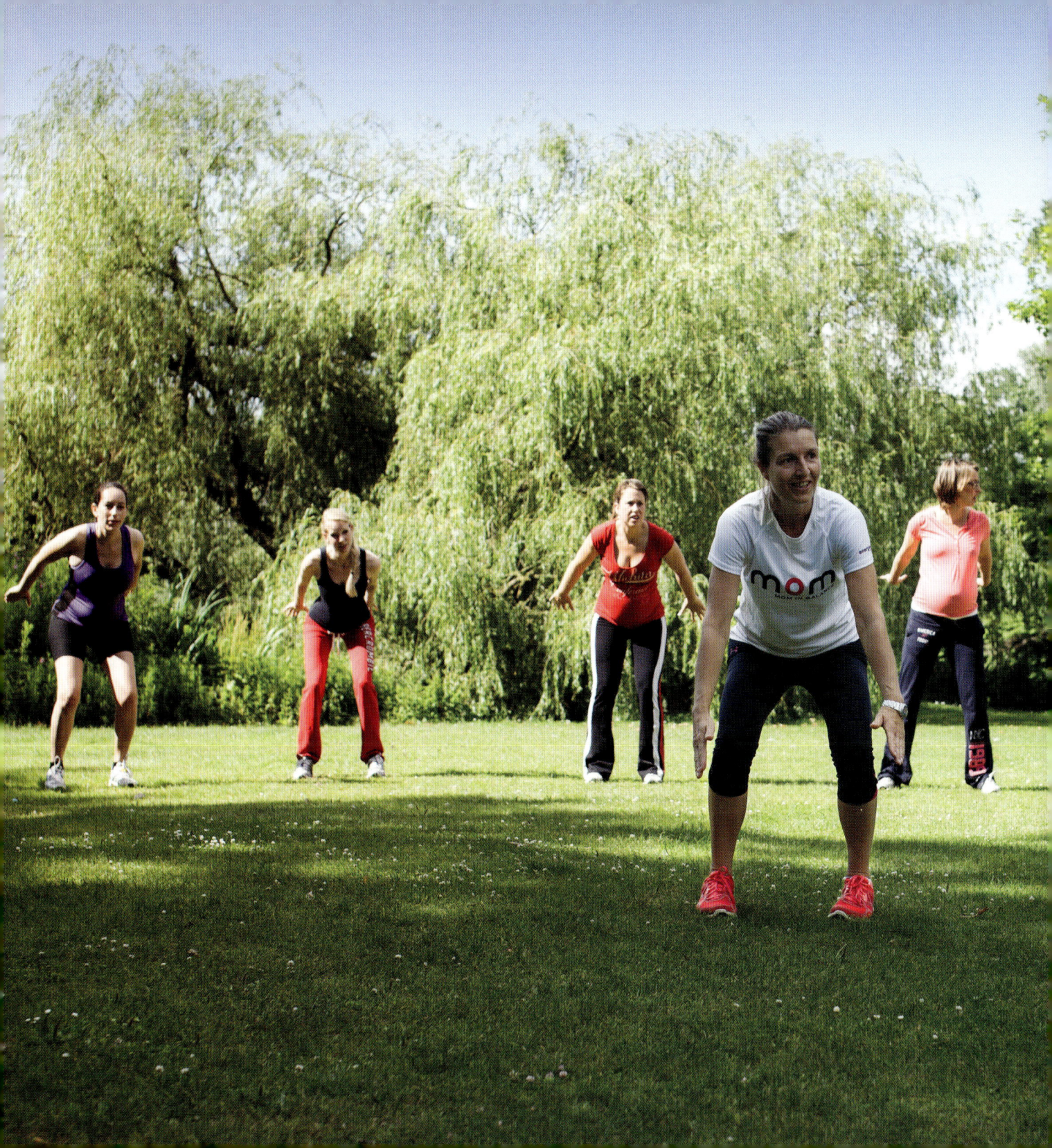

Strong muscles - upper body

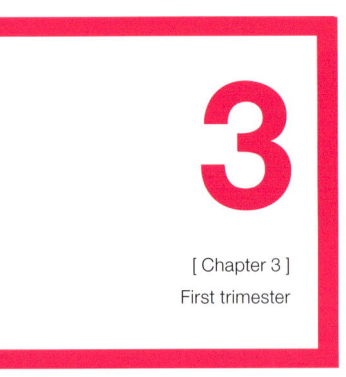

3

[Chapter 3]
First trimester

Most arm exercises are done with a Thera band. This is an elastic belt with which you use your own body resistance to strengthen your muscles. The exercise can be made lighter or heavier by making the belt longer or shorter. You can bring the Thera band along on trips easily as it is very light weight and you can still do your workout wherever you are.

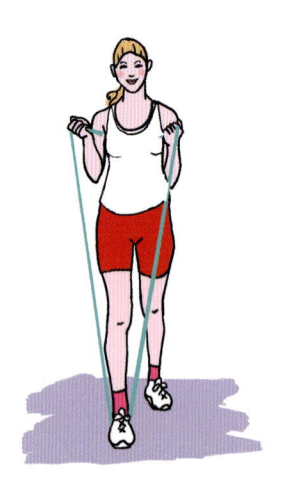

Biceps bend and stretch

This is a good exercise to strengthen your biceps, the front of your upper arms.

1. Stand up straight and place the band halfway under your front foot and hold the band tight at hip height.
2. Bend both arms slowly upwards up to your shoulders and keep your elbows close to your body. The palms of your hands point upwards.
3. Lower your arms again without losing the tension of the band.

Repeat the exercise 10-12 times.

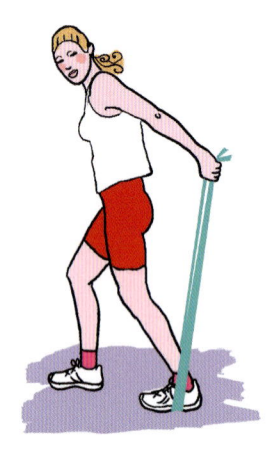

Backward triceps push

This exercise works very well for 'wobbly' arms and strengthens the triceps on the back of your upper arms.

1. Step forward with your right foot and place the band under your back foot. Your knees are slightly bent.
2. Take the band at hip height with your right hand, palm of your hand turned toward the body. Pull the band with a straight arm backwards and return, but keep the tension on the band.

Repeat this exercise with both arms 10-12 times.

Thera-bands are available in the bigger sports stores, but you can also order them online at www.mominbalance.com.

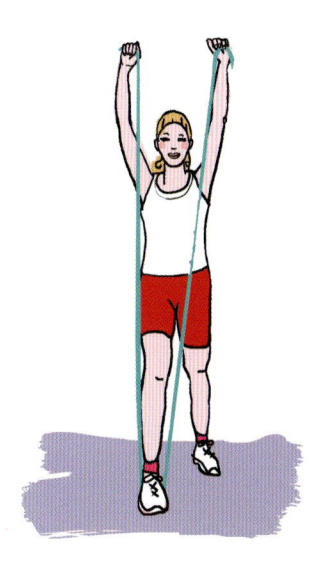

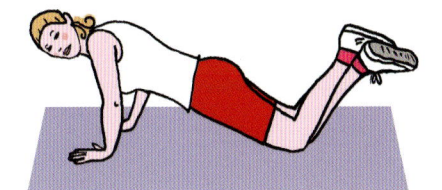

Biceps and shoulders

This exercise strengthens your biceps and gets your shoulders in good shape.

1. Take a big step forwards and place the band halfway under your front foot. Keep your abs well contracted.
2. Keep both ends of the band tight with the palm of your hands down. Bring the band with stretched arms at shoulder height and then stretch your arms in a straight line above your head.
3. Hold this position for 3 seconds and then lower your arms to shoulder height again.

Repeat this exercise 6-10 times.

Push-ups

Push-ups are a complete training for every important arm muscle. A good exercise therefore, to keep your upper body strong.

1. Sit on your hands and knees, with both hands directly below your shoulders on the ground. Keep your knees slightly bent. Keep your abs tightened to prevent tension in the lower back.
2. Bend your elbows and lower your body slowly. Keep your body in a straight line, with your head and shoulders aligned with your spine.
3. Push your body up, until your arms are stretched.

Repeat the exercise 5 times, take 3 seconds rest and then do it another 5 times.

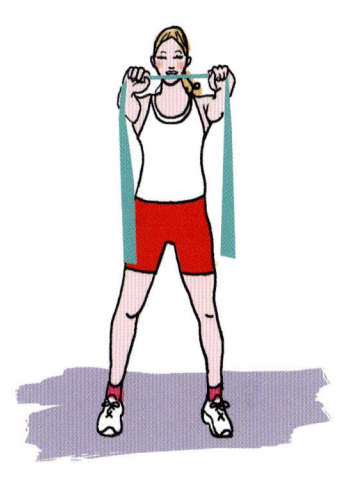

Back and arms

This exercise strengthens your upper back muscles plus the whole length of your arms.

1. Stand up straight with your feet apart so that they are in one line with your shoulders. Keep the Thera band with stretched arms in front of your chest with ca. 15 cm between both hands.
2. Pull the band sideways so that your shoulder blades are pulled towards each other.
3. Go back slowly to the starting position without losing the tension on the band.

Repeat the exercise 8-12 times.

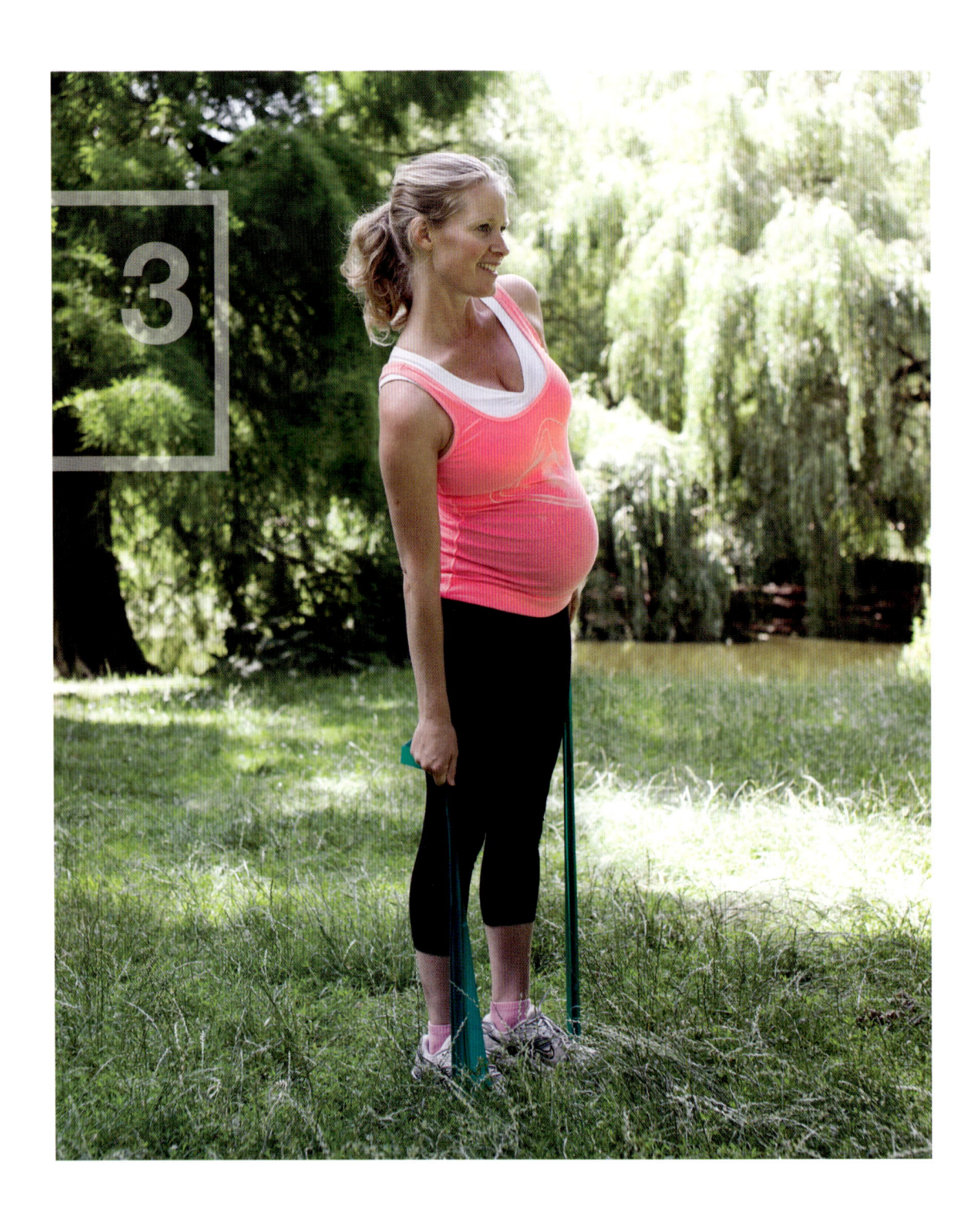

3

Strong muscles - abdominals

During the first trimester of your pregnancy you can exercise your abs like you were used to. Use the following exercises. Strong abs support the pelvis and help in keeping back pain at bay.

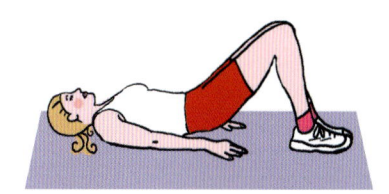

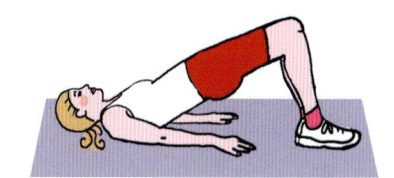

Hips up

To strengthen your core.

1. Lie on your back with both knees pulled up and your feet flat on the ground. Put both arms at your sides, palms down, tighten your abdominal muscles.
2. Press your lower back to the ground, then bring your pelvis up as far as possible and then go back slowly to the starting position.

Repeat this exercise 12 times.

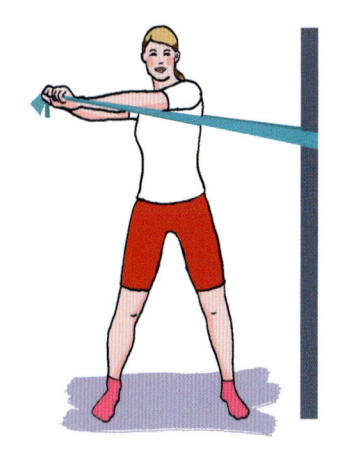

Strong core sideways

This exercise with the Thera band is very effective to strengthen your back and abdominal muscles.

1. Wrap the middle of the Thera band around a pole or doorknob. Stand up with both feet in one line with the hips and keep your knees slightly bent. Hold the double band at the end with both hands.
2. Lift your arms to shoulder height, stretched forward. Pull the band with stretched arms 90 degrees to the right and then come back slowly to the starting position without lowering your arms.

Pull the band 8 times to the right and then 8 times to the left.

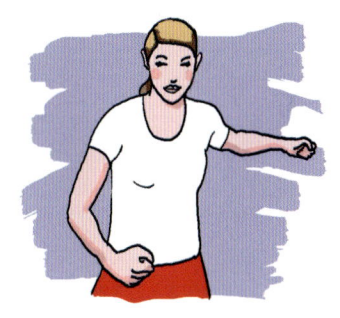

Boxing

With this boxing exercise you train your abdominal muscles and work on a strong and flat belly.

1. Stand sturdy with feet parallel and hip-distance apart and your knees slightly bent. Make fists and draw in your abs.
2. Alternately hit your right and left fist from outside to inside with short hits aiming for your navel. Keep your abs tightened and keep on doing this for 15 seconds.

Repeat this exercise twice.

MOM IN BALANCE

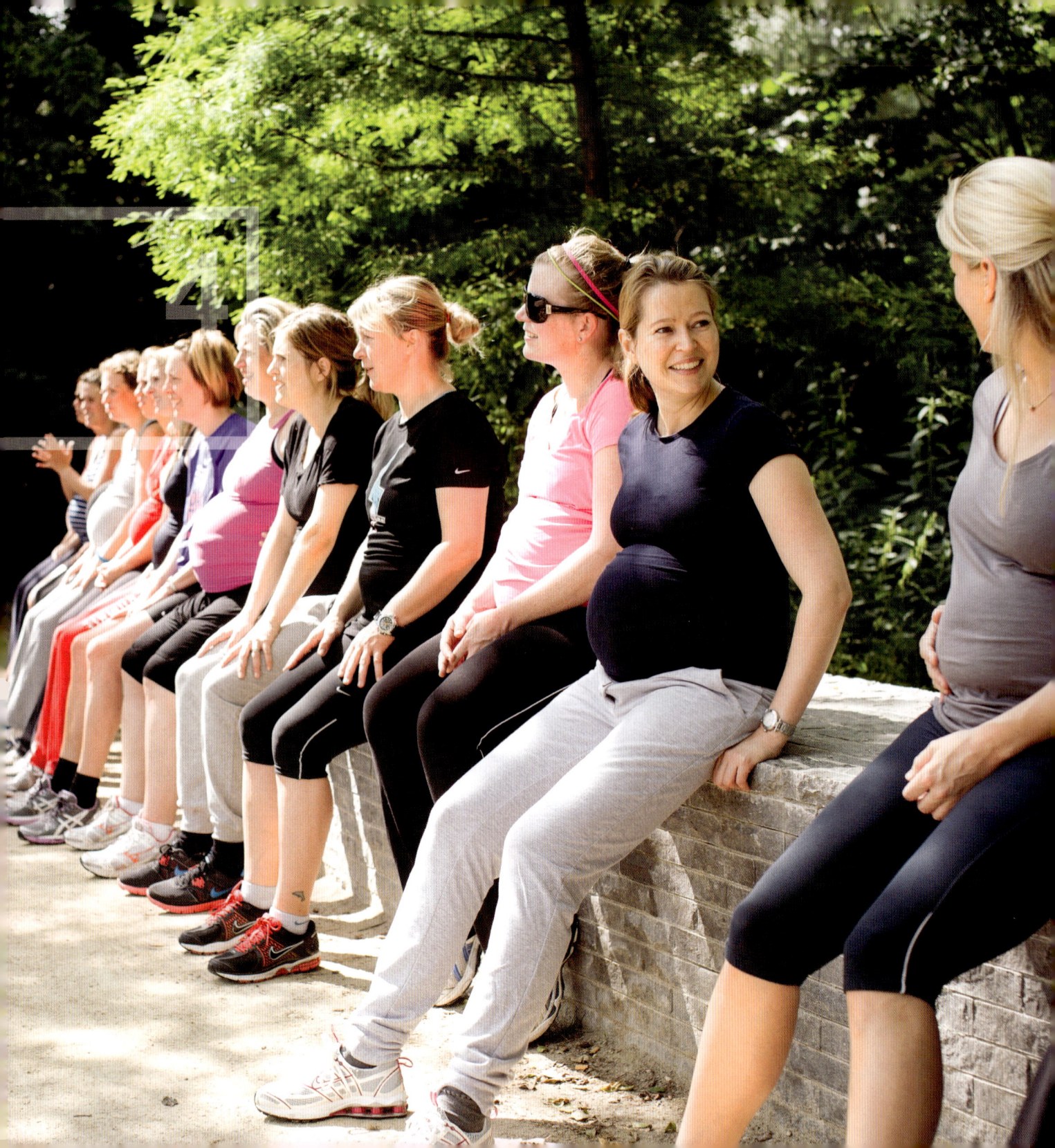

4

[2]Second trimester

week 13 to 27

You got through the first trimester, wonderful! The fatigue and / or morning sickness will slowly disappear now or will be gone already. At the beginning of the second trimester most women feel much better.

Great if you managed to hold on to a sports routine during the first trimester, keep up the good work. For those who didn't get around yet during the first trimester to put on their sneakers: don't panic! It is never too late to start. Especially during the second trimester, when any lost energy has returned, it will be easier to motivate yourself to put on your sports gear.

Physical changes

4

[Chapter 4]
Second trimester

Now that you can actually show a baby is growing inside you, you will need to take certain factors into account when you exercise. Below you will find the most important bodily changes you will experience during the second trimester.

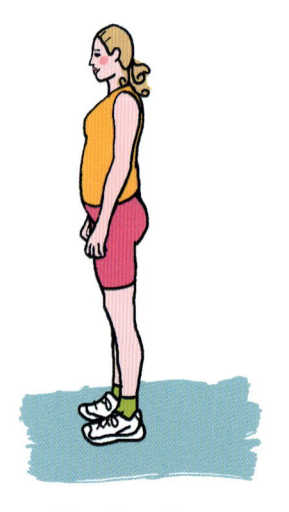

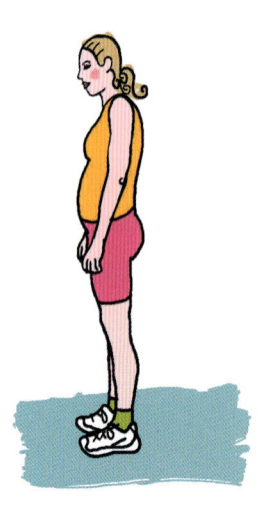

Good posture **Weak posture**

Change of posture
During the second trimester your pregnant belly will start to show. It may take a bit longer for some, but usually when you are at the end of the second trimester, you can be a proud mom to be.

Now that your womb is growing, your centre of gravity will move, pushing your pelvis a bit forward. This will cause a natural hollow in your lower back. So especially now it is important you keep having the right posture.

Posture check
- Stand straight and make your upper body long
- Tilt your shoulders in a V-shape backwards and then easily lower them .
- Keep your knees slightly bent
- Divide your weight as much as possible on both your feet.
- Keep your buttocks neutral below your core.
- Relax your belly (very important), too much tension on the belly may cause pelvic problems.

Flexible joints
Around week 20 of your pregnancy, hormones cause the cartilage and the ligaments which connect pelvic parts to soften.

This will make your pelvis more loose and stretchy, which is good because it will be easier for the baby to come out during labour.

Sometimes the joints in the pelvis become too mobile, causing pelvic problems. This usually happens when the muscles cannot compensate for the increased mobility of the joints. A proper posture and avoiding any heavy burdening will impact those pelvic problems positively. Especially now it is important to strengthen the muscles around your pelvis. When you have pelvic pain problems you can still do a great deal, but you have to find more balance between being active and resting.

Here you will find useful tips for when you feel your pelvis is starting to bother:
- Vary between longer stretches of sitting, standing, lying down and walking. Go for a walk or bike ride regularly.
- Make sure you take time to rest, lie down for a while if you can.
- Don't do too much in one go, but spread your chores over the day.
- Make sure not to keep your legs together tightly, keep your legs a little parted.
- If you like sitting with your legs crossed, that is fine, as long as you do not tighten your leg muscles.
- If the pain worsens, go see a registered pelvic-physiotherapist. He or she can give you even more specific exercises to reduce the problems you have.

The abdominal muscles
As your pregnancy progresses, so does your baby grow, and therefore your belly. To make this possible, the straight abs will part from each other, which is called diastasis. This is perfectly normal and they will go back to their pre-pregnancy position in the period after the delivery.

To find out whether your abs already have parted, you can do the following check: lie down with your legs pulled up. Support your back with a cushion, if necessary.

Place the top of your fingers 2 cm above your belly button, this is the point where the straight abs normally touch each other. Tighten your abs and feel, while exhaling, whether you feel a dent between the two straight abs. If you can easily place two fingers in between the muscles, you have diastasis.

If the straight abs have parted, it is better to stop training them, as this actually makes them move further away. However, you should still train your oblique abdominal muscles.

Your weight during the second trimester
In most cases your appetite has returned by the start of trimester 2. You may however develop specific cravings. Your weight increase will stay in check as long as you exercise regularly and eat a broad variety of healthy food. For tips and advice on nutrition see chapter 5.

Retain fluids
About 75 per cent of the women retain a certain amount of fluids during their pregnancy, mostly around the ankles and feet. Especially when your planned due date will be in the summer, this can be a menace, as with hot weather your body retains even more fluids. To regulate the heat your body has an increased blood circulation and therefore needs extra fluids.

Also after a day during which you have been standing a lot you will notice that you will have thicker ankles in the evening. In most cases there is nothing to worry about. The fluids usually are gone again after a good night's rest.

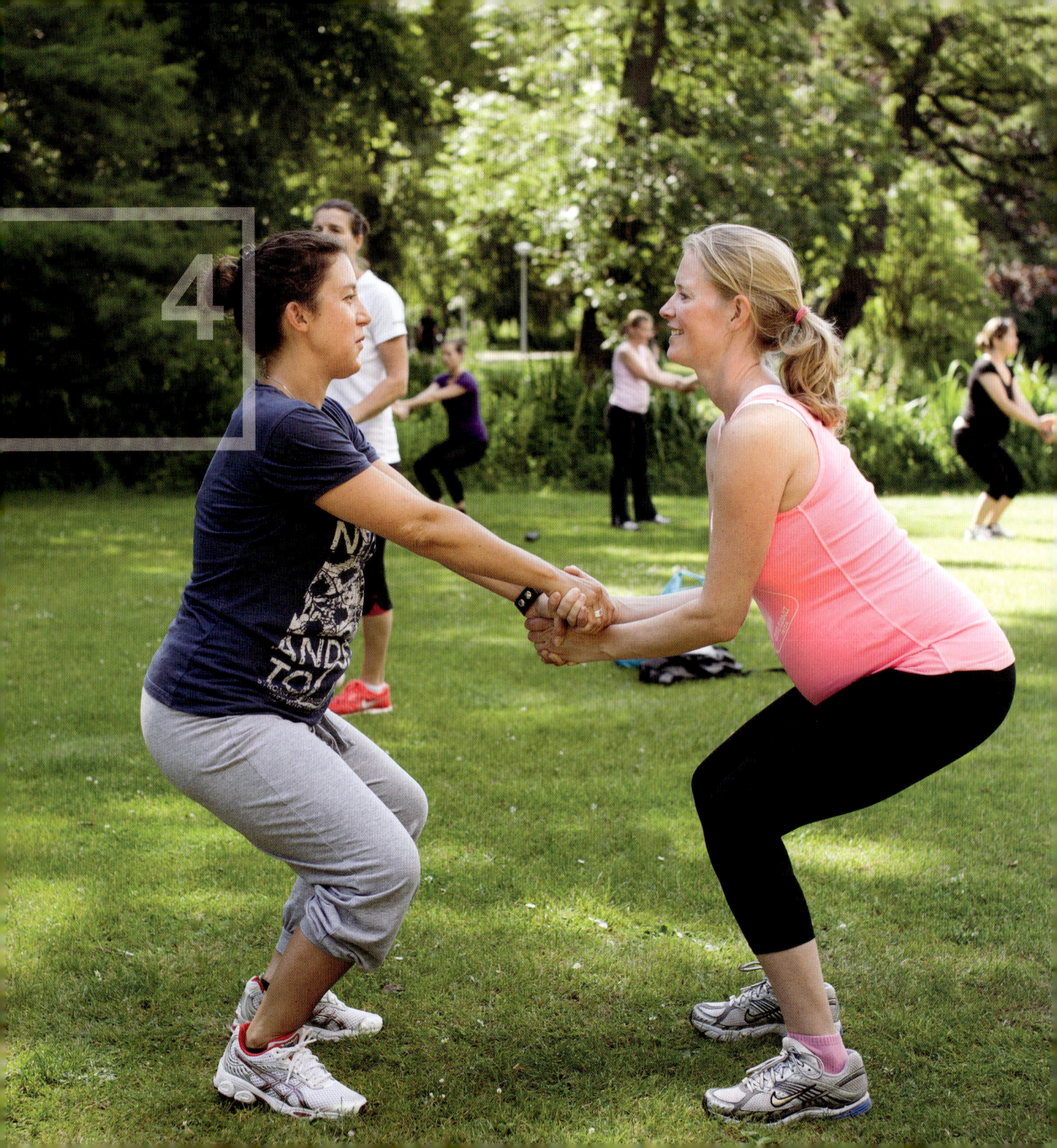

4

These tips help you get through this phase in case you suffer from higher fluid retention:
- Make sure your shoes fit well. Due to the pregnancy and possibly extra fluids your shoes may suddenly be too tight.
- Do not stand in one position for too long. If your profession makes you sit a lot, make sure you go for a walk regularly.
- Put your feet up every time you get the chance.
- Stay active.

Dizziness
During the second trimester you may get dizzy suddenly. The walls of your veins are weaker causing the blood to flow slower. This means you should not get up too quickly, especially after having done your floor exercises, make sure you get up slowly.

Hard stomach
During your pregnancy your womb contracts about every 20 minutes. This keeps it in perfect condition. Usually you don't feel anything, only later in the pregnancy you might start feeling it a bit. During these contractions your belly will feel hard and tense, also called a hard stomach. This can be unpleasant but it is totally harmless for the baby. A firm belly often happens when you exert yourself, but usually disappears when you relax again.

When you are exercising, you may get a hard belly. If that occurs once every now and then, there is no issue, but if they return more frequently, it is better to take a day off. These hard stomachs should not be painful, so do contact your doctor or obstetrician if they do.

Ligament aches
Your uterus is kept in place in the abdominal cavity with ligaments. These ligaments grow with the uterus. This can sometimes be painful, called ligament pains. These ligaments are low in the belly and you can feel the pain in your underbelly and groin. Especially at the end of the second trimester, you may feel these a bit now and then. You can still do your exercises, but you better take it easy for a while, and start your activities after that.

Varicose veins
Developing varicose veins is also a symptom caused by hormonal changes. The hormones change the veins, they become weaker, and can therefore circulate blood less effectively. This can cause blood to accumulate in the veins, which can cause swellings and sometimes also pain, especially at the end of the day. If you suffer from varicose veins, I advise you to stay active. Exercising will make sure your blood flows well and your muscles stay strong. Avoid sitting or standing for too long , and preferably do not cross your legs. If necessary, it can be helpful to wear compression stockings, but not during your workout.

Exercise in the second trimester

4

[Chapter 4]
Second trimester

If you maintained your sporting routine during the first trimester of your pregnancy, you will have no trouble continuing this during the second trimester, as in most cases you will feel much better now. If you stopped doing sports during the first trimester, or if you haven't even started yet, this is the right time!

Physical changes will follow up quickly after each other in the coming trimester. Staying active will help you going through those changes fit and fine and that you can keep all the pregnancy issues under control.

Now that you have reached the second trimester you may have noticed already that the hormones are doing their job: you sometimes feel your head is all cloudy, you can't think straight anymore. This may cause you to bump into things or drop things. There are a few reasons for this 'clumsiness'. First of all, the hormones: relaxine causes your joints -and particularly your pelvic- to become more loose. That is why you don't stand so sturdy like you used to. Secondly, the growing weight of your belly and breasts make it harder to hold your balance. When doing activities with lot of sudden moves, like tennis for instance, you will have to watch out, you don't want to spend the rest of your pregnancy on the couch with an injury.

Mom in Balance Pregnancy workout

Exercising with other pregnant ladies is motivational to keep up your own sports routine. Next to meeting other great people of course! So look for options in your neighbourhood, or -if you happen to have a pregnant friend- set dates to go for a walk or a swim. During the second trimester you can start the Mom in Balance sports workouts, where cardio training is combined with stretching and muscle strengthening exercises. Check www.mominbalance.com to see whether there are Mom in Balance workouts in your city.

Putting together your Action Plan
Fill out your action plan here for the second trimester of your pregnancy.

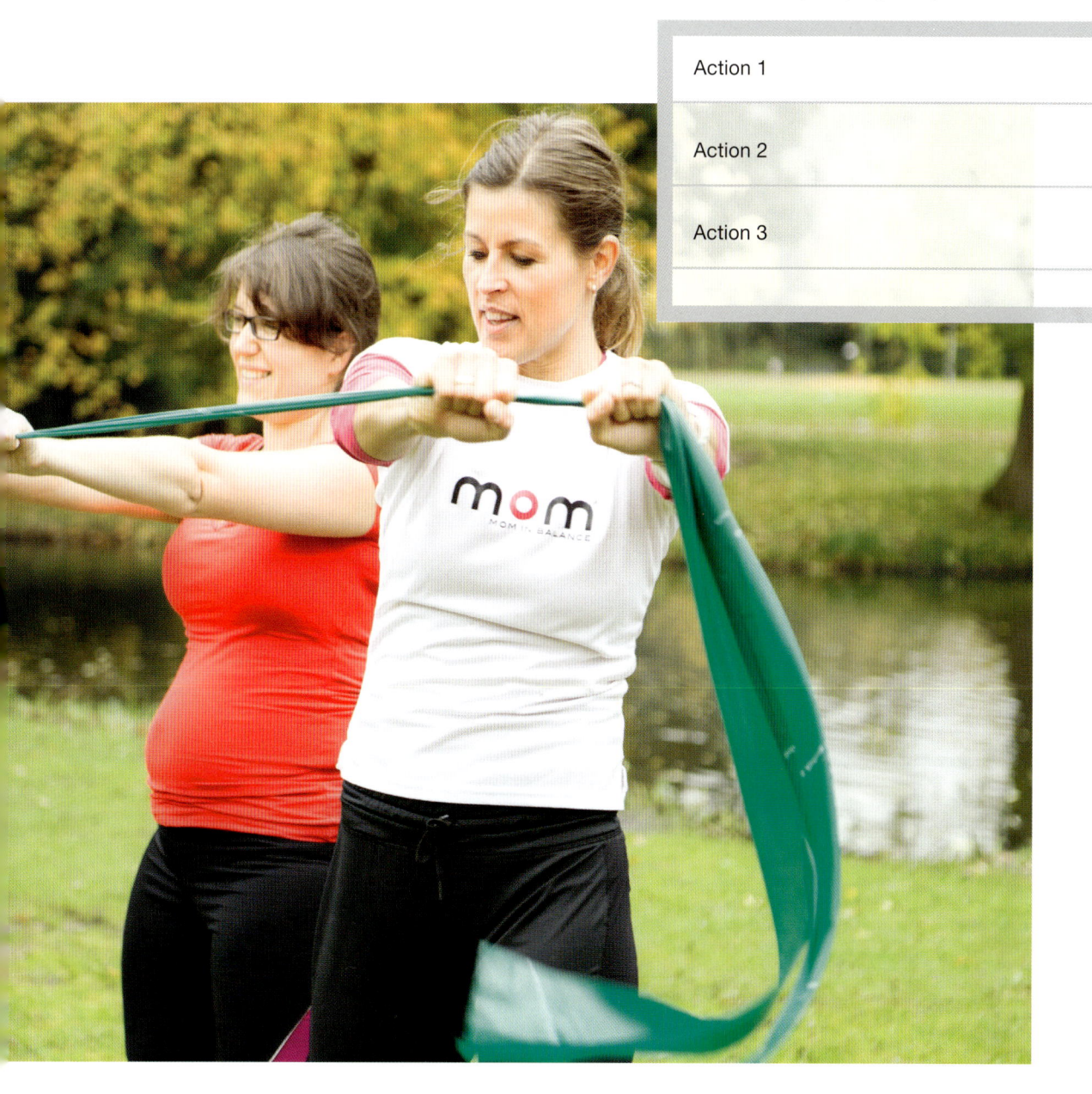

Action 1	
Action 2	
Action 3	

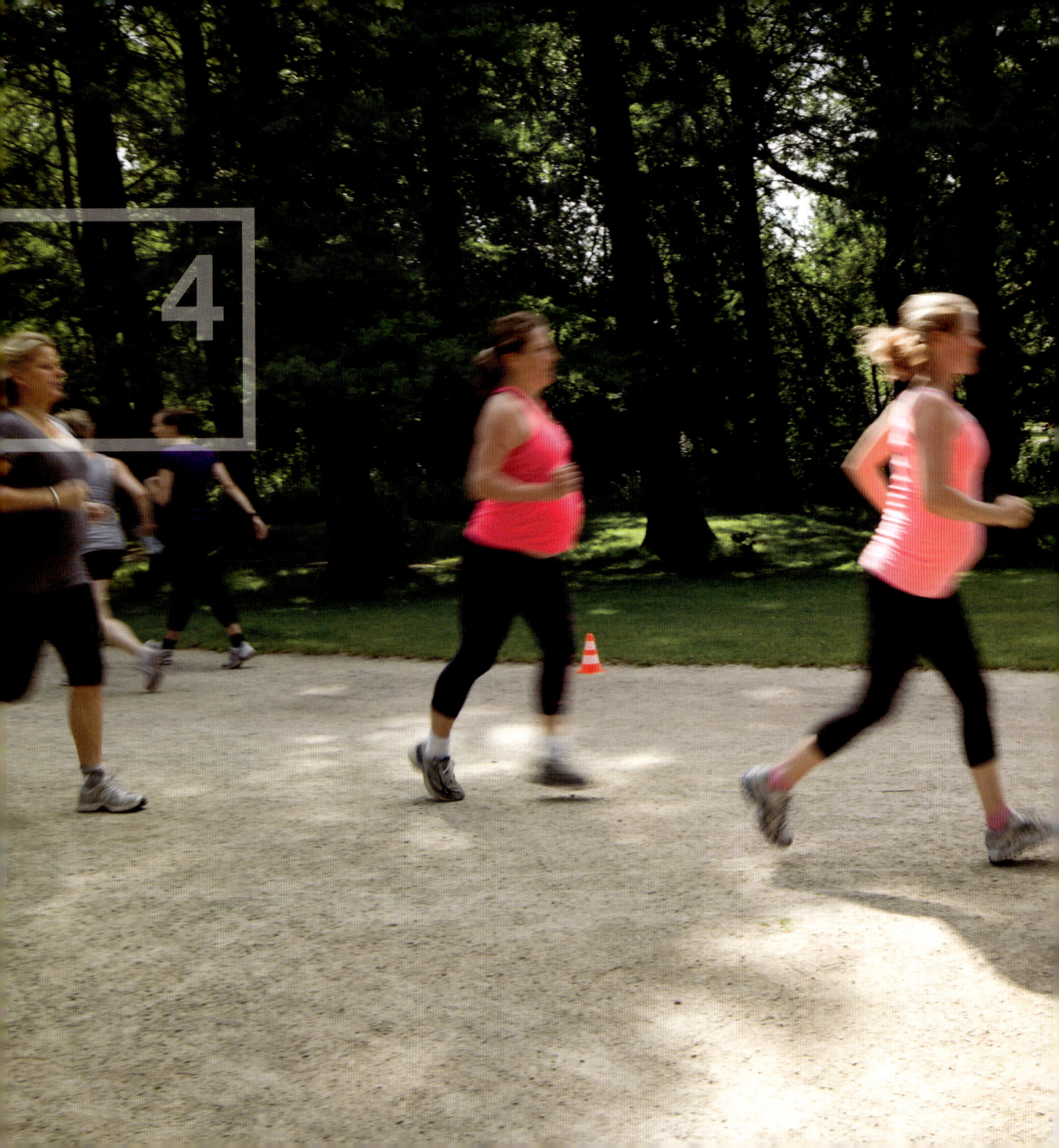

4

Cardio-fitness

As you probably feel much better now, it will be easier to plan your cardio workout . Try to make time for this. You will notice it will give you an energy boost which you can use very well the coming months.

A few tips that may be useful during your workouts in the second trimester:

1. As I already indicated earlier, your physical balance will be less now. So keep facing forward and train on a flat surface.
2. Replace sports that do not feel comfortable anymore by sports you still think are pleasant to do. If jogging becomes too hard, change to a brisk walk or start swimming instead.
3. Remind yourself you are not doing your exercises to lose weight, but to stay healthy during your pregnancy. So do not try to work off those extra kilos you are gaining right now.

The next training schedules may bring variation to your workout.

FLYING START

"I could look forward all week to the Mom in Balance workout on Saturday mornings in the park in Amsterdam, funny enough nearly always with the morning sun shining brightly. Doing sports with other pregnant women with expert guidance gave a flying start to the weekend: physically all recharged, but also during the stretching exercises discussing the latest developments or getting some advice from the 'fat bellies' on prams, nutrition and baby essentials.'

Hanne, Mom in Balance-participant

Keep going! - beginning athlete

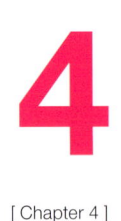

4

[Chapter 4]
Second trimester

If you are just starting to build up your sports routine during this trimester, I am very happy you do. Even when you start now, you can still enjoy all the benefits an active pregnancy will offer. You do need to build it up slowly though.

Walking
It is more important that you keep up your 3-days a week routine, than doing a workout for one long stretch at once. That is why I recommend you start with a simple cardio workout, which you can easily fit in your busy schedule. For most people going for a walk is the simplest way to get into action. You can do it everywhere and you don't need much.

Walking schedule
The first 2 weeks try walking 3 times a week for 10 minutes. Then slowly build it up to 15 minutes per walk. If you find this easy, proceed with the walking program for the starting sportswoman, chapter 3, page 37.

Swimming
Swimming is relaxing and you train all your muscles at once. An ideal cardio workout to start with. Use the swimming program underneath:

Swimming schedule
For the warming up, always start with a 5-10 minutes swim in a slow pace, 2-4 laps of 25 meters.

Swim 2 laps, rest 1.5 minute
Swim 4 laps, rest 2 minutes
Swim 2 laps, rest 1.5 minute
Swim 4 laps, rest 2 minutes
Swim 2 laps, rest 1.5 minute
Swim 4 laps, rest 2 minutes
Swim 2 laps in a slow pace

This workout, during which you swim 22-24 laps, takes about 25 minutes. If this distance is a bit much for you the first few times, do only half the number of laps and build it up slowly to 30 minutes max.

Keep going! - trained athlete

If you managed to hold on to your sports routine, then I will give you new variations to keep on walking, jogging or swimming. During the second trimester you can also continue with a combination of the three activities: walking/jogging, swimming and biking.

Swimming
If you need an alternative for jogging or if you are looking for a workout which is easy on your joints, this is a good time to jump into the pool. Swimming gives your body a total workout.

Swimming schedule
For the warming up, always start with a 5-10 minutes swim in a low pace, 2-4 laps of 25 meters.

> Swim 4 laps, rest 2 minutes
> Swim 8 laps, using a board, rest 3 minutes
> Swim 6 laps, rest 3 minutes
> Swim 4 laps, using a board, rest 2 minutes
> Swim 4 laps, rest 2 minutes
> Swim 2 laps in a slow pace

This workout, during which you swim 30-32 laps, takes about 30 minutes. Total workout of 30-32 laps is 750-800 metres.

Walking/jogging
If you still enjoy jogging, please keep it up, and use the jogging schedule in chapter 3, page 39.

If you wish to continue your walking routine, it's good to start the walking program below. You will vary between a relaxed pace and a fast pace here.

Walking Schedule
Start with a 5 minute easy walk to warm up your muscles. Then walk 5 minutes at your normal walking pace.

During the next 16 minutes you alternate a 1 minute fast walk with 3 minutes easy walking, but keep up a steady pace. End your walk with a 5 minute easy walk to cool down your muscles. To avoid injuries, I recommend doing some stretching exercises after the walk.

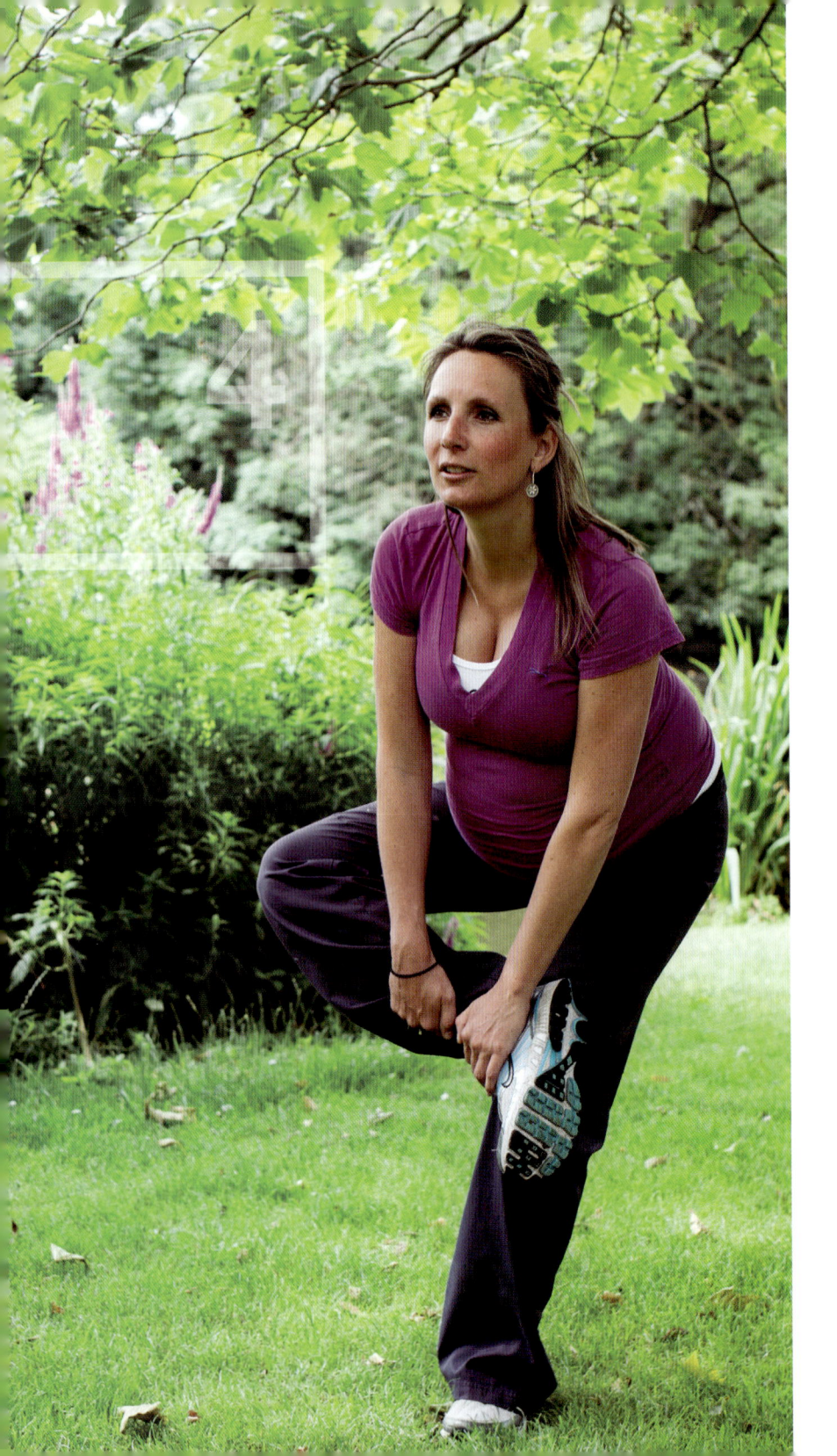

Stretchen

Hopefully you started your stretching exercises already during the first trimester and has it become second nature to stretch every now and then. When you managed to get to that point, you will probably stand up straight better and feel more comfortable in your changing body - very good!

Don't panic if you haven't reached that point yet, because during the second trimester you can still start with the program. By keeping your muscles flexible you will avoid lower back pain, cramped calf muscles, a bad posture and other problems as much as possible, so do get into action right away with those stretching exercises. Also do the stretching exercises of the first trimester (page 41).

Below here you will find different stretching exercises for the upper and lower body, and you can start right away.

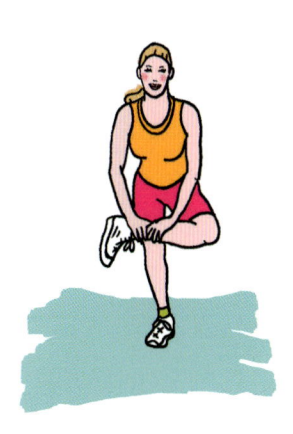

Gluteal muscle (buttocks) stretching

With this exercise you stretch the deep-seated glutes very well.

1. Stand up with your feet at hip distance and your knees slightly bent.
2. Bend your left leg and cross your left foot over your right leg, just above the knee.
3. Lower your right leg as far as possible. You will feel it stretch in your left hip, left buttock and at the top of your left thigh.

Hold the stretch for 10 seconds and then switch legs.

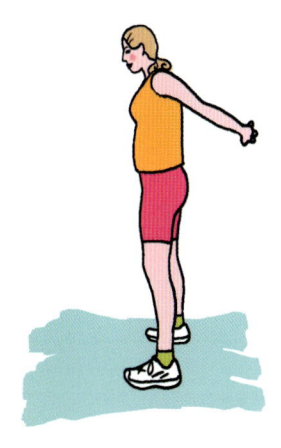

Pectoral (chest) muscle

With this exercise you stretch especially your pectoral muscle, the larger muscles at the front of the chest.

1. Make sure your back is straight and that your head and neck are in line with your spine.
2. Hold your left hand with your right hand around the back. Stretch both your hands slowly backwards, keeping your arms straight. This way your shoulder blades will be pushed together and your chest comes forward automatically.

Hold the stretch for 10 seconds.

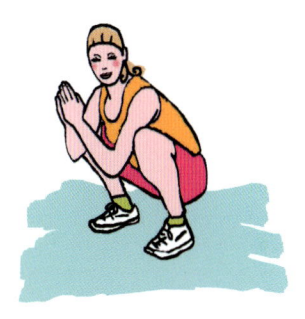

Lower back stretching

With this exercise you stretch and relax your lower back. If your lower back is bothering you during the day, I recommend you do this exercise more frequently.

1. Stand up with your feet a little wider than your hips and keep your abdominal muscles tightened.
2. Lower your knees slowly and sit as low as possible. Try to keep your feet flat on the ground.

Hold the stretch for 10 seconds and repeat this twice.

Strong muscles - legs and buttocks

4

[Chapter 4]
Second trimester

Now that you are into the second trimester of your pregnancy, you probably notice why it is so important to be physically strong. Pregnancy is a big physical challenge. If you already started with muscle strengthening exercises during the first trimester, your legs will probably be a lot stronger, which will help you carry the extra weight of your belly.

It is also important to make your upper body stronger. Strong arms make lifting easier, and that can be handy if you already have a kid running around. Now that your abs are becoming less strong, and the weight of your belly increases, it certainly is convenient to have a strong upper body. Next to that a strong back helps you keep a nice straight posture despite the extra weight in the front.

The following exercises are probably not intensive enough to give you a bodybuilding look, but they sure will make you feel stronger.

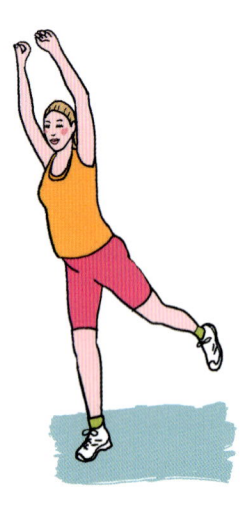

Leg lift - backwards

With this exercise you make your glutes, your lower back and the back of your hips and hamstrings tighter and stronger.

1. Stand up straight with both knees slightly bent.
2. Tighten your abs to support your back and tighten your glutes.
3. Bring your left leg backwards still with your glutes tightened. At the same time, stretch your arms above your head.
4. Slowly come back to the starting position.

Repeat this exercise 8-12 times with both legs.

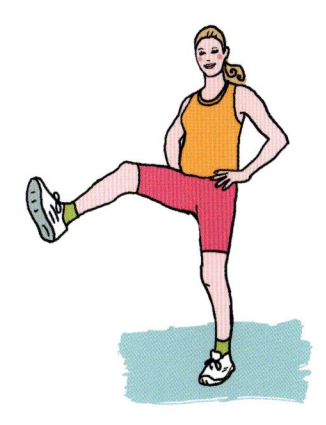

Leg lift - forwards

This exercise strengthens your quadriceps, hamstrings and butt plus you train your hip muscles.

1. Stand up straight with your feet together and if necessary, use a chair for support.
2. The left leg knee is slightly bent. Move your right leg forwards to the point that it still feels comfortable.
3. Hold this position for 3 seconds and then return to starting position.

Repeat this exercise 8-10 times with both legs.

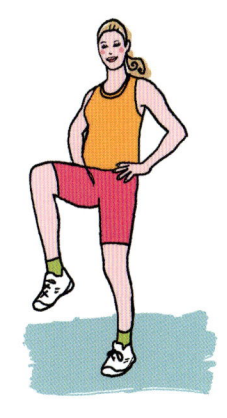

Knee lift - standing

This exercise loosens your hips plus front upper leg muscles like the quadriceps.

1. Stand up straight and keep your abs contracted.
2. Lift your right knee until your foot is as high as your left knee.
3. Return to the starting position and repeat this with your left leg.

Repeat this exercise 10 times.

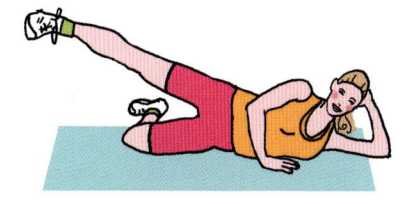

Leg lift- lying down

Your thighs will gather a small layer of fat during your pregnancy. With this exercise you will make sure your legs stay nicely shaped.

1. Lie down on your left side with your head supported by your forearm, with your body forming a straight line and keep your abs tight.
2. Bend your left leg in a 45 degree angle and tilt your pelvis slightly forward.
3. Lift your right leg a little, stretched, and lower it again. Tighten your glutes at the same time.

Repeat this exercise first 15 times with your right leg, then 15 times with your left leg.

MOM IN BALANCE

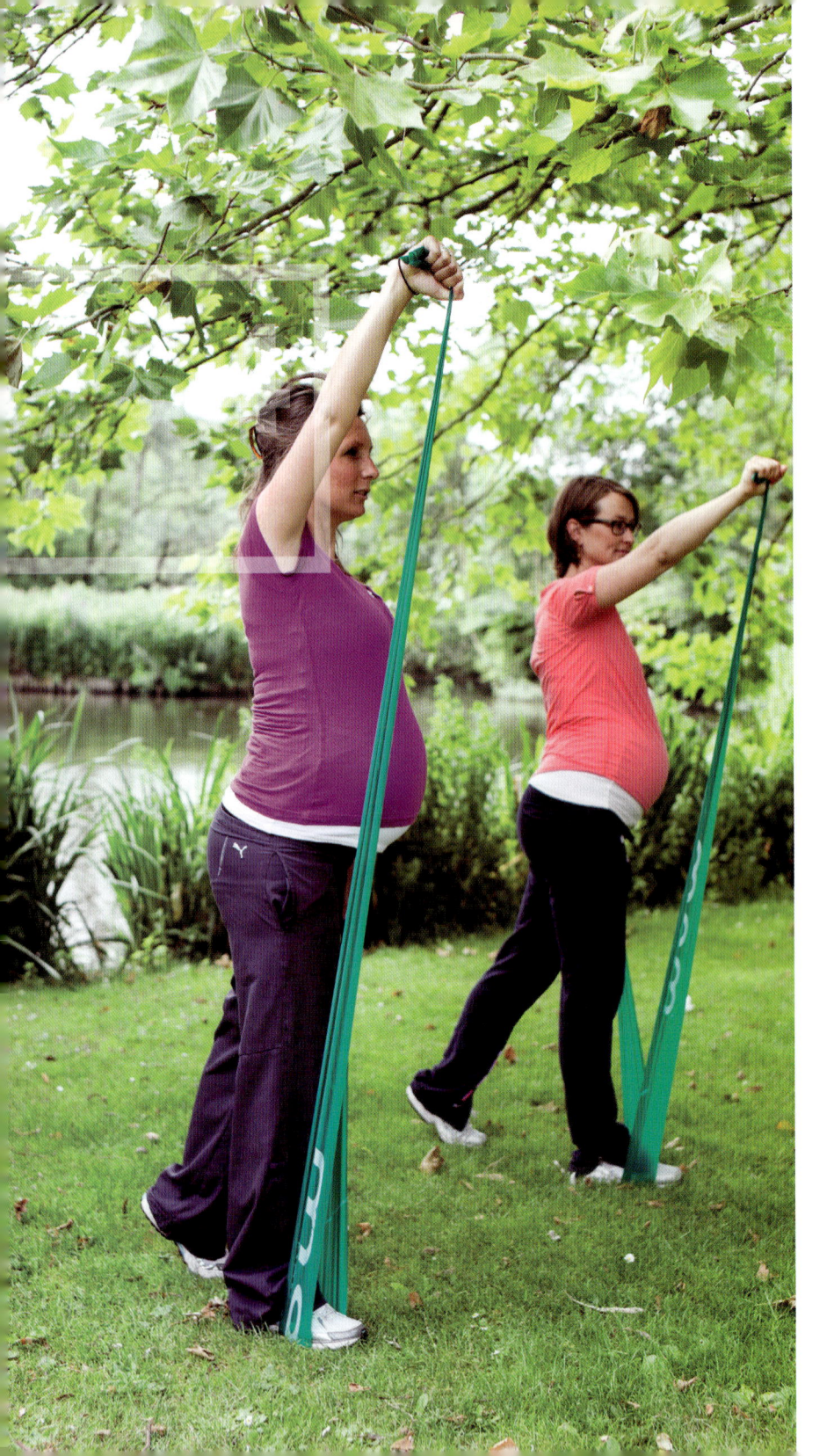

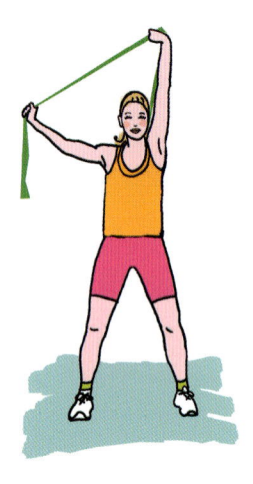

Strong upper arms

This exercise strengthen your upper arms, shoulders and upper back. It also stimulates a straight posture.

1. Place your feet parallel shoulder-distance apart, with your knees slightly bent.
2. Hold the Thera band with both hands, with ca. 20 cm space between both hands and lift your arms stretched above your head.
3. Hold your left arm stretched upwards and pull with your right arm the band down towards your waist.
4. Return to starting position and switch to your left arm.

Repeat this exercise 12 times.

Strong muscles - arms

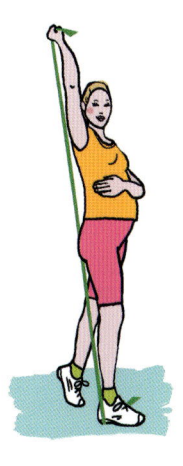

Triceps training

With this exercise you train your triceps at the back of your upper arms.

1. Stand up straight with your abdominal muscles slightly tightened.
2. Stand and put your weight with your right foot on one end of the Thera band and hold the other end with your right hand.
3. Lift the band with your right hand around the back in a straight line, as far as possible, while your back foot is on its toes.
4. Lower the band while your elbow keeps pointing upwards.

Repeat this exercise 8 times with both arms.

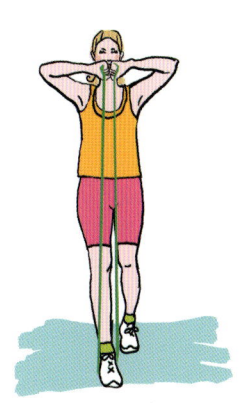

Strong shoulders

This exercise keeps your shoulders in good shape and you will strengthen your upper body.

1. Take a step forwards and put the middle of the Thera band under your right foot.
2. Take the band at both ends and keep your abs tightened.
3. Move your hands to each other and pull the band up at shoulder height, with your elbows pointing outwards.
4. Pull up the band a bit, and lower it again to shoulder height.

Repeat this exercise 8 times

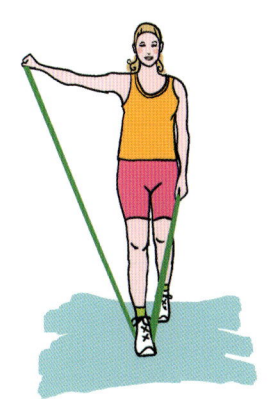

Great arms

With this exercise you train the whole length of your arms and shoulders.

1. Take a step forward and wrap the Thera band halfway the front foot.
2. Hold the band with both hands and pull it with your right hand with stretched arm sideways to shoulder height.
3. Lower the band again but keep the tension on the band.

Repeat this exercise 8 times with both arms.

MOM IN BALANCE

Strong muscles - pelvic floor

4

[Chapter 4]
Second trimester

As your pregnancy progresses, there will be a period where your pelvic floor muscles will endure extra pressure. These muscles support your urinary channel, bladder and womb and they will absorb all the extra pressure on your underbelly during physical pressure.

During your pregnancy your muscles will weaken as a result of all the hormonal changes. The same will happen with your pelvic floor. From above the pressure on the pelvic floor will increase considerably because of your baby growing. This may cause an imbalance and you may suffer from incontinence or subsidence. It is therefore important that you exercise your pelvic floor muscles during your pregnancy to prevent these problems. It will also help you to feel and train the pelvic floor muscles more easily after your delivery.

How can you find your pelvic floor muscles

The focus of these exercises during the pregnancy is mainly on feeling, not strength. You must be able to tighten your pelvic floor muscles, but also be able to relax them. So it is important to practice both.
How do you tighten your pelvic floor muscles?

- Try to pull in your urethra, vagina or anus a bit.
- Try as if you were to prevent breaking wind
- Go and sit down on a rolled up towel or empty hot water bottle (this way you increase the pressure on your pelvic floor) and try to pull up your vagina.
- Put your hand against your perineum, the piece of skin between your vagina and anus and try to pull it in.
- Try different ways: lying or sitting down or standing up
- Make sure your belly and butt do not tighten as well.
- Put the focus on feeling, not strength.

Train your pelvic floor every day

Exercising your pelvic floor muscles

Try to exercise your pelvic floor muscles daily. Because you pay attention to tightening as well as relaxing during these exercises, you cannot overtrain your pelvic floor muscles.

Because of a good and optimal relaxation the pelvic floor functions better, on top of that relaxing is also important for the delivery. Here are some examples to exercise your pelvic floor.
- For the general condition of the muscle: tighten for 50% and hold for 4 seconds, then rest for 8 seconds, repeat this 3 x 10
- Exercises for more control: when you exhale slowly, tighten the pelvic floor 60%, then rest for 8 seconds, repeat this 3 x 10.
- Focus on feeling: tighten the muscle from 25 to 50 to 70%, then rest for 8 seconds, repeat this 3 x 10.

Important to know for your pelvic floor exercises during your pregnancy.

- After each time you tighten your pelvic floor, always release it in one go, not in phases.
- Your pelvic floor will not function better by doing the exercises more powerful, it is much more important to have control and that you feel it well.
- Do not shorten the resting period after each tightening, because relaxing is just as important to get the pelvic floor working well.
- Never train it when you are walking or jogging.
- Try to exercise your pelvic floor daily with 3 x 10 repeats each time. E.g. do it while brushing your teeth, taking a shower, having breakfast or watching the news.
- Never exercise your pelvic floor while urinating, you may increase the chance to an inflammation of the bladder.

Using your pelvic floor during your daily activities

Because of tissue becoming weaker during your pregnancy and the increasing weight of your belly, it is important to actively use your pelvic floor during heavy physical activities. Try to teach yourself to tighten your pelvic floor during lifting, pushing or pulling moments. Also while coughing or sneezing you could tighten your pelvic floor.

Registered pelvic physiotherapist

Despite all the exercises and advice it can happen that you still face problems. E.g. incontinence, subsidence, or pelvic pain. If you have problems, make sure you get In touch with a registered pelvic physiotherapist.

4

[Chapter 4]
Second trimester

Strong muscles - abdominals

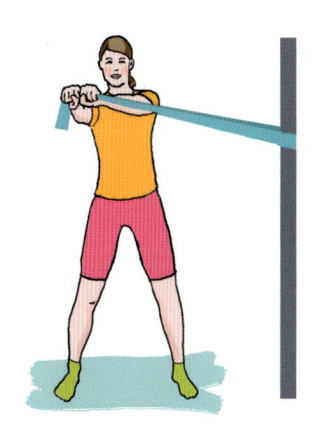

During the second trimester you will concentrate more on the oblique abdominals. If you can already feel the straight abs part (see page 55), stop training these. The oblique abdominal muscles you can train all the way until the end of your pregnancy.

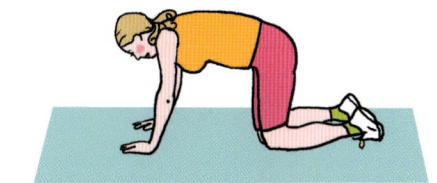

Strong core
To strengthen your back and abdominals.

1. Wrap the middle of the Thera band around a pole or doorknob. Stand about a meter from the pole with both feet parallel at hip-distance and keep your knees slightly bent, so that there is sufficient tension on the band. Hold the double band at the end with both hands.
2. Lift your arms at shoulder height, stretching forward. Hold your arms stretched and pull the band with short jerks again and again, further to the right. Do this for 10 seconds.

Repeat this exercise twice to the left and right side.

Contracting your stomach
This exercise will help you get a good posture.

1. Get down on hands and knees. Put your hands at shoulder distance with your elbows slightly bent and your knees below your hips. Keep your head aligned with your spine and look at the ground, without pulling your chin towards your chest.
2. Relax your abs and pull your belly-button inwards as far as possible.
3. Tighten your abs for 10 seconds and then slowly relax.

Repeat this exercise 3 times.

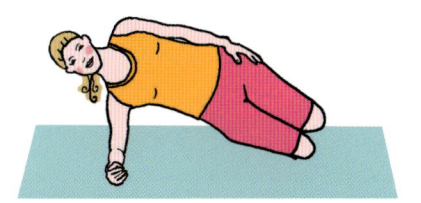

Outer abdominal muscles
With these exercises you strengthen your outer oblique abs.

1. Lie down on your right side. Lean on your right underarm and bend both knees in a 90 degree angle backwards. Keep your upper legs in a straight line with your upper body.
2. Lift your hip as far as possible and keep this position for 5 seconds. Then slowly lower it again.

Repeat this exercise 3 times with both hips.

MOM IN BALANCE

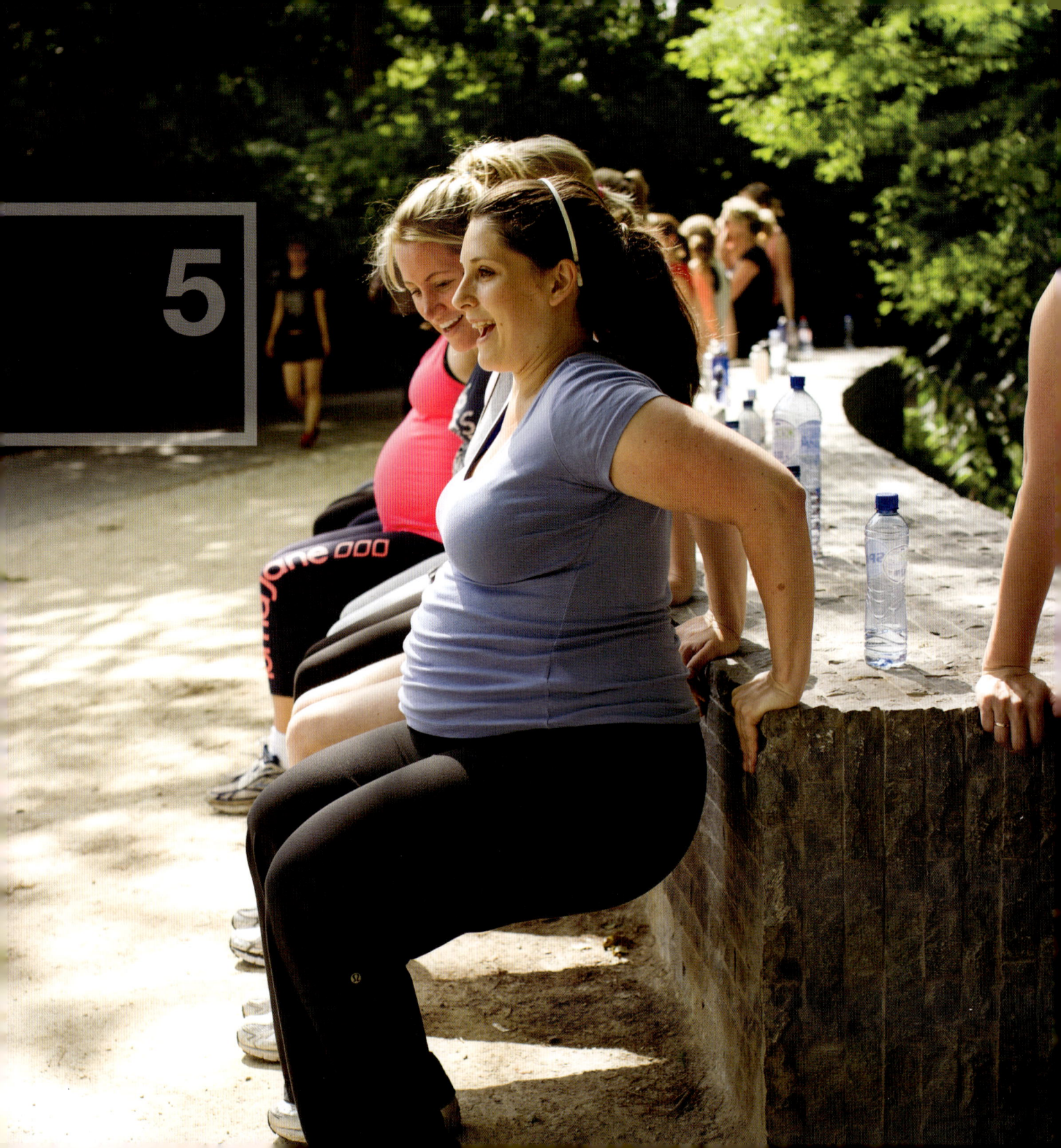

5

[3] Third trimester

week 28 to 42

You have reached the last trimester of your pregnancy, which runs from week 28 to week 40-42. During the 6th month of your pregnancy your belly will have grown considerably and you can now proudly show you are pregnant. Especially now that your body is actually changing, you want to keep on feeling well and you probably can use some extra energy. To keep the last months of your pregnancy as pleasant as possible, I strongly recommend to keep on doing exercises and watch what you eat.

If possible and you have planned pregnancy leave you can enjoy your time off. Even if you feel very heavy by that time, staying active will keep you feeling good. Next to that it is very important that during the last weeks of your pregnancy you take enough rest. After all, you want to be fit and relaxed when you go into labour. The nice thing of pregnancy leave is that you can do a workout during the day now too.

From my own experience I know it takes quite a bit of discipline to keep on doing your exercises all the way till the end, but I also know that it will make the last months of your pregnancy very pleasant and positive.

Physical changes

5

[Chapter 5]
Third trimester

Your body is clearly changing now and carrying around those extra kilos is already a workout on itself! So every credit goes to you for making an exceptional achievement already. During the last trimester of your pregnancy your baby will grow to its full birth weight. So it is quite nice when your body is in top shape. Below you will find the various bodily changes you can expect during the last months of your pregnancy.

Changing posture
When discussing the second trimester I already mentioned that maintaining the right posture is very important. The more your belly is protruding, the more hollow your lower back will be. This can easily cause lower back pain, especially when you have to stand a lot. Do the posture check regularly, which I described on page 54, this will help prevent lower back pain a great deal. Next to that, your growing belly and may your pelvis are becoming more and more lose, and make you start to waddle. Especially when the baby has engaged it can be harder to lift your feet properly. That may cause your walks to be shorter. Give in to this and listen to your body. You can still do everything that feels good and comfortable, but adjust your activities when needed.

Out of breath
During the last months of your pregnancy you will notice you will loose your breath more easily. When you are panting after you walked the stairs, you feel as if your condition has reduced to zero. However do not let this scare you - all the hard work of the last months has certainly not been in vain.

Now that your baby is growing rapidly, your womb has become about 20 times as big. You can feel it pushing into your ribs. Your lung and breathing capacity already was impacted by the progesterone hormone, and now your lungs don't even get enough space do their job properly. This is why you have a hard time catching your breath. Particularly for super fit pregnant women this may be quite a shock. The moment the baby is engaged you will feel you get your breathing space back. Walking upright also helps to give your lungs more space.

Increased heart rate
I mentioned before that during the first trimester of your pregnancy your heart beat is rising because of all the extra blood your body needs for the baby to grow healthily. When your pregnancy advances your heart beat will increase even further: during the first trimester your heart

Tips to prevent calf cramps

To prevent nightly calf cramps, you can do the following exercise before you go to bed: first stretch the calf muscle by setting one foot in front of the other with heels flat on the ground and stretch the calf on the back leg. Then with your feet close next to each other first lower your knees and then make yourself long again, and stand on your toes. Repeat this exercise at least 5 times. This way you stimulate the blood circulation in your calf muscle. Should the cramp hit again, stretch your leg and pull your toes towards you. This will relax the calf muscle.

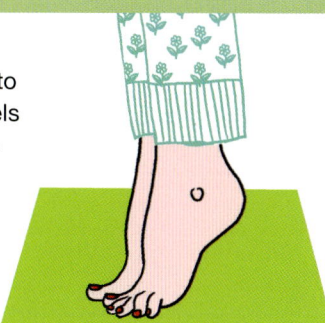

beat will be about 15 beats per minute higher than before you got pregnant. In combination with the extra weight you are carrying now, your body needs more oxygen. That is why it is getting increasingly harder to keep the same intensity in your sports activities. Don't consider this a sign of failure! Your body is working just as hard for that lower intensity, so your condition remains at the same level.

Weight increase

During the third trimester you gain on average about 5 kg. Rest assured, this will not all end up on your hips and butt. Your baby is going to hold on to fat more during the last months, to be able to survive better outside your belly. At the end of your pregnancy you probably have gained about 10-15 kg. You will be surprised how big your belly can get. Continuing to do your workouts will definitely help you carry this extra weight better. Staying active will also help you In bouncing back to you pre-pregnancy shape faster after the delivery.

Leg cramps

When you finally found a comfortable position and are fast asleep, you may, especially towards the end of your pregnancy- suddenly be brutally woken up by heavy calf cramps. These nasty cramps - which sometimes also occur during sports - or during sex- happen in general more often when you're pregnant. This is caused most probably as pregnant women can suffer from a calcium and magnesium deficiency.

A cramp attack may be quite painful, but is nothing to worry about. If you get these cramps a lot, make sure you get enough calcium. After consulting your obstetrician or doctor you may take calcium- or magnesium supplements.

MOM IN BALANCE

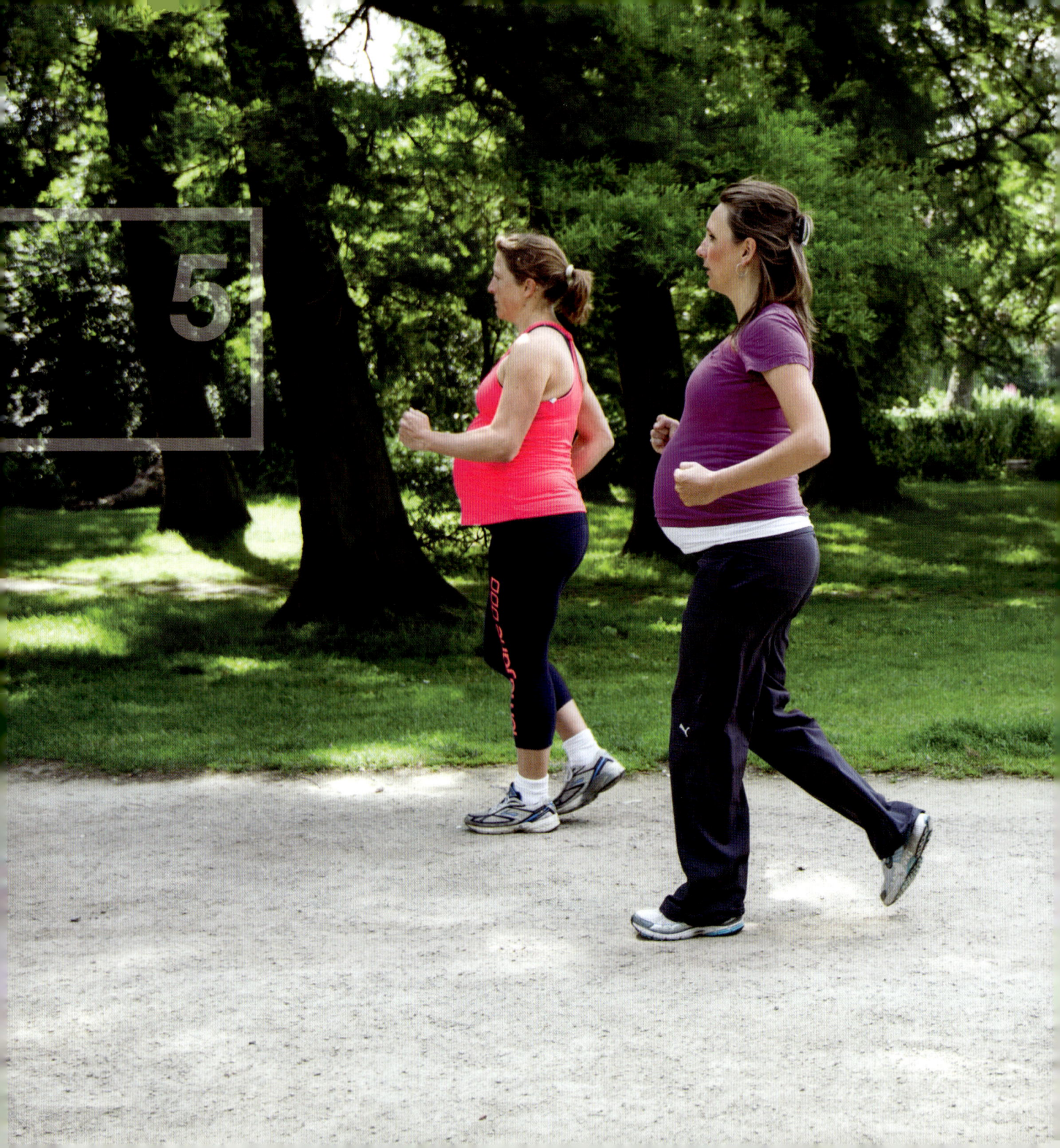

5

Workouts in the third trimester

Action 1
Action 2
Action 3

By staying active and eating healthily during the last trimester you will keep your condition in shape and you will prevent excessive weight gain during the last few weeks. This way you will be well prepared for the delivery.

Different studies show that continuing to do your exercises until the end of your pregnancy can help shorten the delivery time (Clapp, 2002). By doing sports you at least have developed endurance which will help you get through the delivery better. More than enough reasons to stay active, also during the last trimester of your pregnancy.

Your action plan
Fill in your plan of action above for the third trimester of your pregnancy. Check the tips on page 34 again to stay motivated also during those last months.

I FEEL GREAT

"I'm now in my 40th week of my pregnancy, and I can recommend everybody to keep on staying active. I have had a perfect pregnancy without notable problems. I am still doing my exercises now, every day, and I feel great."

Margriet, Mom in Balance-participant

Cardio-fitness

[Chapter 5]
Third trimester

Now even every activity you do, no matter how small, will help keeping up your heart condition and gives the endurance you will need when the big day comes. Next to that, staying active during the last months is the best weapon against pregnancy aches and pains like back pain and fatigue.

However, you do need to adjust your sports activities those last few months. With your joints getting more flexible, the chance of injuries increases, so sports that involve a lot of sudden movements should really be avoided now until after the delivery. During the last trimester cardio workouts are a great way to keep your physical condition in top form, the various exercises you find in this chapter.

Although during these last weeks you are not so jumpy and fast as you used to be, your body is working overtime right now. This is a good moment to admire your hardworking body for the work it has been doing the past few months. Just keep in mind that your physical possibilities are limited at the moment but that your current condition is only temporary and you will be rewarded soon.

When you passed the 40 weeks, you can still do your exercises after consulting with your obstetrician or doctor. A daily walk can help switching your thoughts to something else and make the waiting a bit more pleasant. But I do advice not to do total marathon walks or an enormous load of exercises.

CARDIO-FITNESS

Use the different cardio schedules for the starting and experienced sports woman

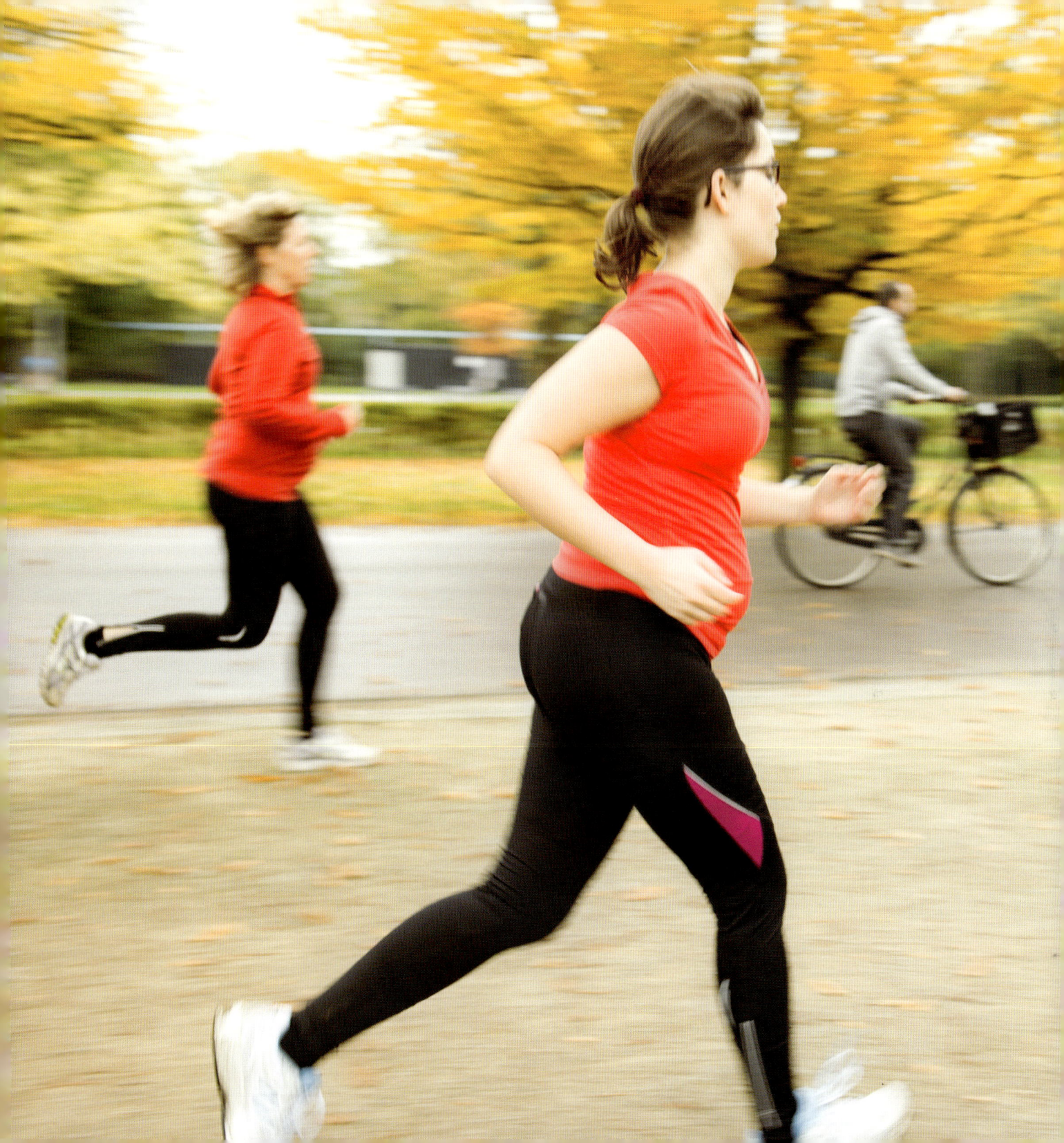

Almost there! - beginning athlete

[Chapter 5]
Third trimester

If you haven't been able to exercise during the first and second trimester, it's not too late and you can still get into action! But always consult with your obstetrician or doctor.

This is not the moment to fire away a complete sports program at your newly formed body, but during the third trimester you can still perfectly well start with the exercises and cardio workouts. But do take it slowly!

Walking
Walking is a good exercise to start with in the third trimester. It gives you lots of energy and it will make sure your physical condition will keep in shape. Use the walking program below to build it up slowly.

Walking schedule
During the first two weeks try to get into a routine of a daily 10 minute walk. If you've managed to do that, go to the walking program for the starting sportswoman, described in chapter 3.

Swimming
Swimming is also a good activity to start with. Your joints will hardly be burdened and you feel nice and light in the water.

Swimming schedule
To warm up, always start with a 5 to 10 minute swim in a slow pace, 2-4 laps of 25 meters.

Swim 2 laps, rest 2 minutes
Swim 2 laps, rest 2 minutes
Swim 4 laps, rest 3 minutes
Swim 2 laps, rest 2 minutes
Swim 2 laps, rest 2 minutes
Swim 2 laps in a slow pace

This workout, during which you swim 16-18 laps lasts ca. 20 minutes.

Almost there! - trained athlete

If you have been taking group classes at the gym or if you participate in the Mom in Balance Pregnancy Workout, you can continue doing so as long as it feels good.

Especially now it is very important to listen to your body, so do adjust if necessary, the intensity of your workout.

Walking and jogging
Walking is still one of the best activities to keep on doing. So if you wish to make a real workout of your walk, continue the program which you started during the second trimester. If you still enjoy jogging, it is fine to continue to do so. But do make sure you do not wear yourself out. You will find out soon enough when it is time to switch to a brisk walk. Now that your body is working very hard during the last trimester you can easily lower the intensity of your workouts, with your condition staying in shape.

Walking schedule
Start with a 5 minute easy walk to warm up your muscles.
Then walk for 5 minutes in a pace you would normally walk.
The next 16 minutes you switch between 1 minute fast walk and 3 minutes relaxed walking, but do keep up a steady pace. End your walk with a 5 minute easy walk to cool down your muscles again. To prevent injuries, I recommend doing some stretch exercises after your walk.

Cycling
If you want some variation in your workouts, cycling offers a very good cardio workout for the last trimester. On the bike you still have enough room for your belly and it can be the solution if you suffer from lower back ache. If your pelvis is bothering you, it is better to walk or swim. And do make sure you lower your speed if you get hard stomachs during cycling.

Swimming
During the third trimester swimming is a great cardio workout. You feel nice and light in the water. For variation you may try using flippers. You will get more speed easier and will not get tired that soon. Furthermore it strengthens your legs and ankles, which you can use well during the delivery. Also your arm muscles will be well trained by swimming.

Swimming schedule
To warm up, always start with a 5 to 10 minute swim in a slow pace, 2-4 laps of 25 meters.

Swim 4 laps, rest 1 minute
Swim 6 laps, rest 3 minutes
Swim 4 laps, rest 1 minute
Swim 6 laps, rest 3 minutes
Swim 2 laps in a slow pace

This workout, during which you swim 24-26 laps, will take about 25 minutes. Total workout of 24-26 laps = 600-650 meters.

Flexible muscles

5

[Chapter 5]
Third trimester

Especially during those last few months you probably have become familiar with little problems like back ache, insomnia and retaining fluids. But you hopefully also discovered that cardio workouts and muscle strengthening exercises reduce many of these ailments. Stretching muscles will also help you prevent these issues and prepare you for the delivery.

I recommend to keep on doing the stretching exercises mentioned in the first and second trimester chapters. Stretching exercises which are particularly suitable for the third trimester can be found below. It Is time to double your effort to do your stretching exercises. You don't have to do all stretches every day, but if you manage to do at least 5 stretches every other day, you will have a great benefit during the delivery.

If you don't find the energy to plan a whole workout, stretching is a perfect alternative and a good focus for your exercises. It's a relaxed way to keep your muscles mobile.

Mobile muscles: legs, back and neck

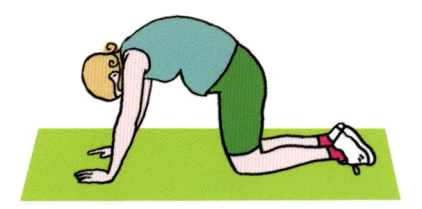

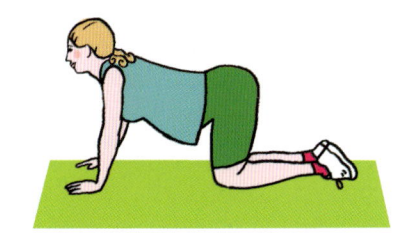

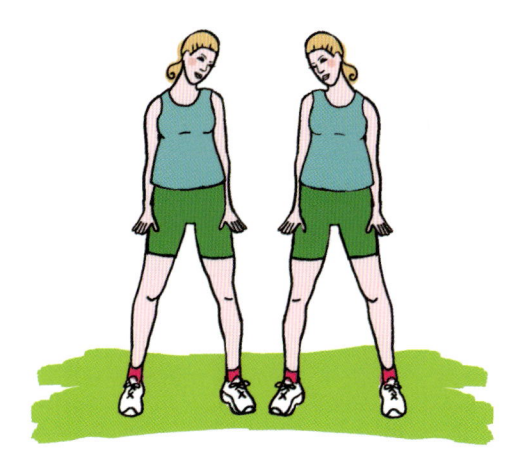

Thigh stretch

With this exercise you stretch the inner thigh. A good exercise to prepare you for the delivery.

1 Sit on the ground with legs bent, the soles of your feet against each other and your knees outwards. Keep the soles together and place your hands lightly on your knees.
2 Keep your back straight and tighten your abdominals a bit.
3 Press your knees with the help of your inner thigh muscles to the ground. Do not bounce them.
4 With your knees as low as possible, hold that position for 10 seconds, then bring your knees slowly upwards.

Repeat this stretch twice.

Cat stretch

With this exercise you will stretch most large muscles in your back. This exercise can be very relieving for lower back aches.

1 Get down on your hands and knees. Keep your head and neck relaxed and face the ground.
2 Make your back round slowly by pulling in your abs and to push the curve of your spine upwards.
3 Hold the stretch for 10 seconds and then lower your back again.
4 Then make your back hollow by lowering your belly and lifting your head.
5 Hold the stretch for 10 seconds then move your back upwards again to a relaxed position.

Repeat this stretch twice slowly.

Neck stretch

This is a very nice stretch which relaxes your neck muscles.

1 Stand up straight with your feet under at hip distance. Relax your shoulders.
2 Start the stretch by lowering your chin slowly to your chest. Hold this stretch for 3 seconds.
3 Then turn your head slowly from left to right and hold the stretch on both sides for 3 seconds. Then turn your head back to starting position and face forward again.

Repeat this series 3 times.

MOM IN BALANCE

Strong muscles - legs and buttocks

5

[Chapter 5]
Third trimester

Now that your belly is getting bigger and bigger, doing muscle strengthening exercises may become quite a challenge. But it will be very beneficial if you manage to continue your workouts. Especially during your delivery and the first weeks after you will be glad you did!

The following exercises will also be fairly easy to do during the third trimester. They are less intensive than the exercises during the first 2 trimesters, making them easier to sustain. If you still feel fit after completing these workouts, you can also keep on doing the exercises from trimester 1 and 2.

Especially when you are nearing the end of your pregnancy, it can be nicer to do a few exercises several times a day instead of one long workout. Make sure you are at ease before the delivery starts. Best of luck, you're nearly there!

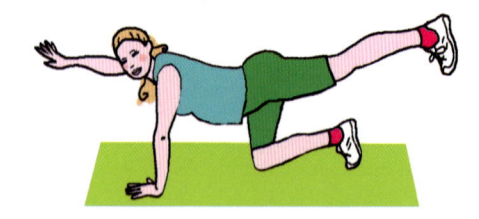

Balance

This exercise helps to improve your basic stability. Next to that it strengthens your joints and makes them more flexible plus you also train your thigh muscles.

1. Get down on your hands and knees.
2. Tighten your abdominals. Stretch your right arm straight forward and hold your left leg backwards. Try to keep both as straight as possible.
3. Hold this position for 3 seconds and then return to your hands and knees again.

Repeat this exercise 3 times with each side.

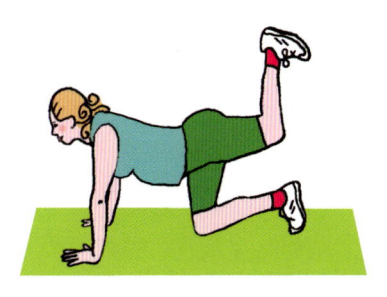

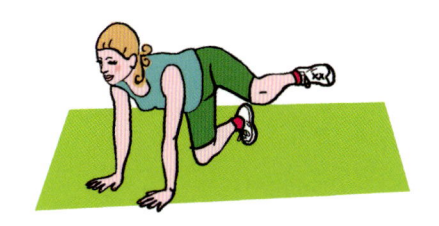

Strong hips

This is a good exercise for the stretch muscles in your hip.

1. Get down on your hands and knees and keep your back straight.
2. Tighten your abs and glutes.
3. If you feel more comfortable leaning on your underarms, please do so.
4. Lift your left leg with your knee bent.
5. Lift the upper leg very slowly 5 cm and then lower it again. Come back to hands and knees.

Repeat this exercise first 5 times with your left leg, then with your right leg.

Thigh lift

With this sideways move you train your outer thigh muscles.

1. Get down on your hands and knees. Keep your back straight and tighten your abdominals to support your lower back.
2. Lift your left leg sideways with your leg keeping a 90 degree angle. Hold this position for 2 seconds.
3. Then return slowly to hands and knees.

Repeat these exercises first 5 times with your left leg, then with your right leg.

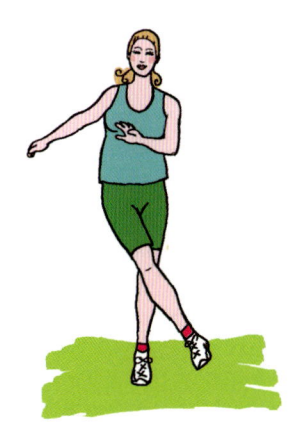

Front side swing

Strengthen your hip muscles with the swing on the front side.

1. Stand up straight with your knees slightly bent and your abs tightened.
2. Lift your right leg and swing your stretched leg over your front side from left to right.
3. Swing 6 times with your left leg from left to right.

Repeat this exercise but then 6 times with your right leg.

MOM IN BALANCE

5

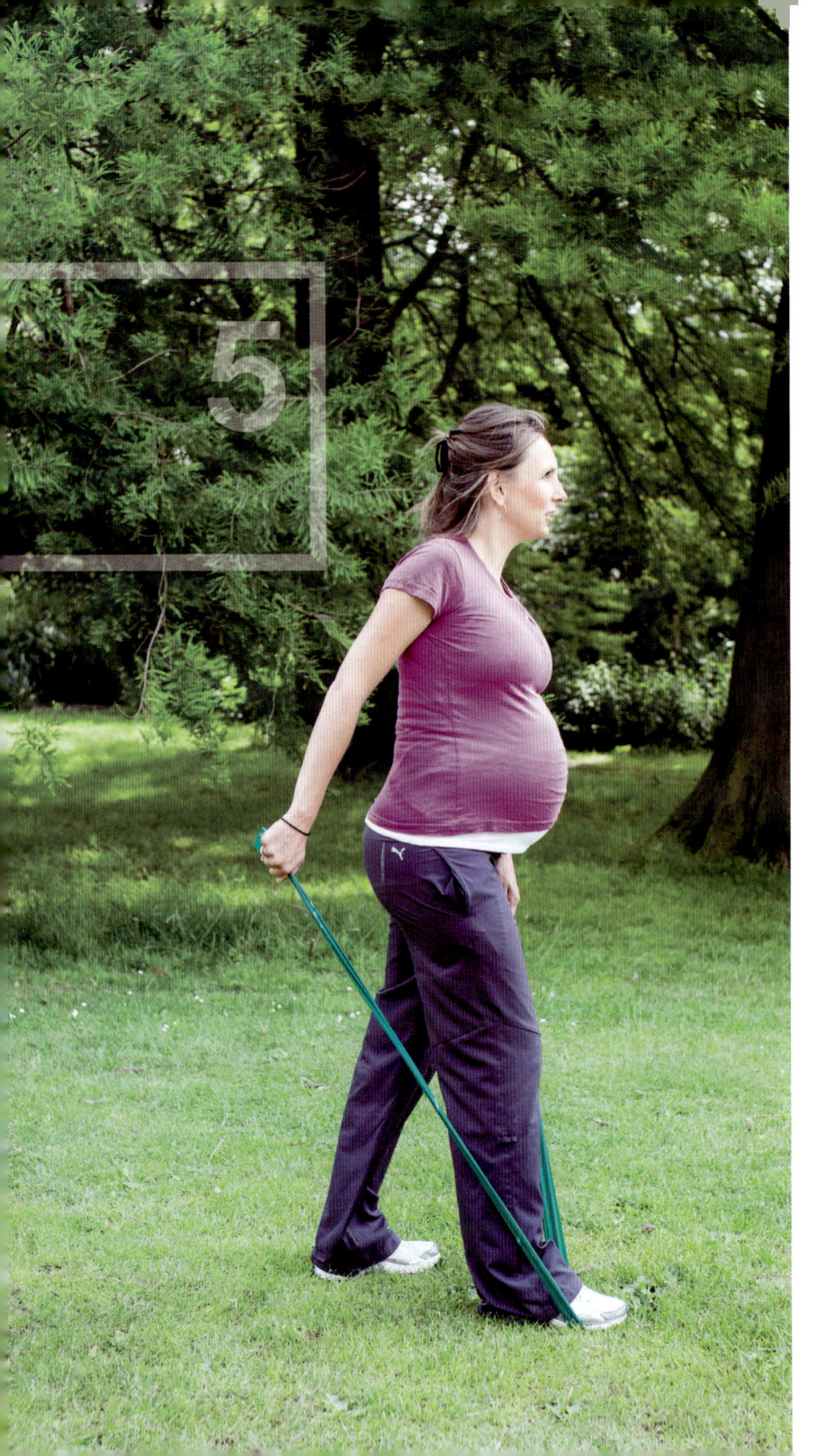

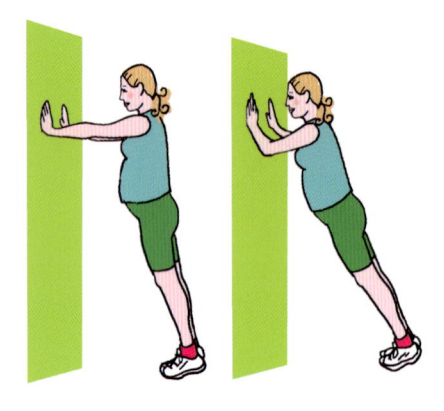

Firm breasts

With this exercise you strengthen all your upper body muscles, especially the muscles under your chest. So a great exercise for firm breasts!

1. Stand about half a meter from a wall facing the wall, with your feet at hip-distance apart. Keep your knees slightly bent.
2. Lean forward and put your hands flat on the wall. Bend your elbows and move towards the wall with your chest.
3. Tighten your chest-muscles and push yourself away from the wall to starting position.

Repeat this exercise 10 times.

Strong muscles - upper body

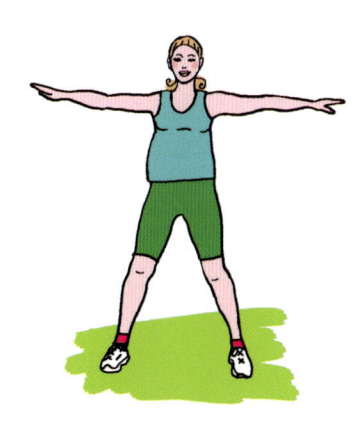

Arms spread

With this exercise you strengthen the length of the top side of your arms.

1. Stand with your feet a little wider than hip-distance. Contract your abs.
2. Spread both arms stretched outwards. Hold this position for 10 seconds and then lower them slowly again.
3. If you wish to make the exercise a little harder, keep your arms stretched and make short up and down movements.

Repeat this exercise 5 times.

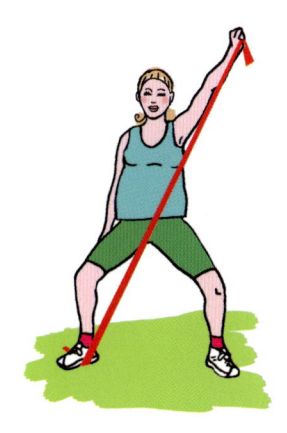

Super squat

This workout strengthens your shoulders and upper back. You also train your upper legs at the same time.

1. Stand with your feet a little wider than your hips. Your feet point outwards. Wrap the thera band halfway under your right foot and hold a long piece of band in your left hand.
2. Lower your buttocks into a squat position and pull the band with your left hand into the left upper corner.
3. Slowly lower the band again but make sure you do not lose the tension on the band.

Repeat this exercise 8 times with both arms.

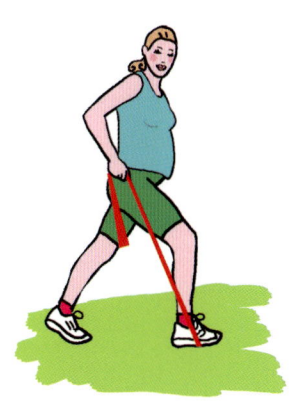

Elbows high

This exercise is meant for the muscle running from your neck to your shoulders.

1. Take a step forward with your right leg and keep your abdominal muscles tightened. Wrap the band halfway under your front foot.
2. Take the band with your right hand and pull the band backwards towards your hip, while lifting your elbow.
3. Make sure there is sufficient tension on the band. Then stretch your arm slowly.

Repeat this exercise first 8 times with your right arm, then with your left arm.

MOM IN BALANCE

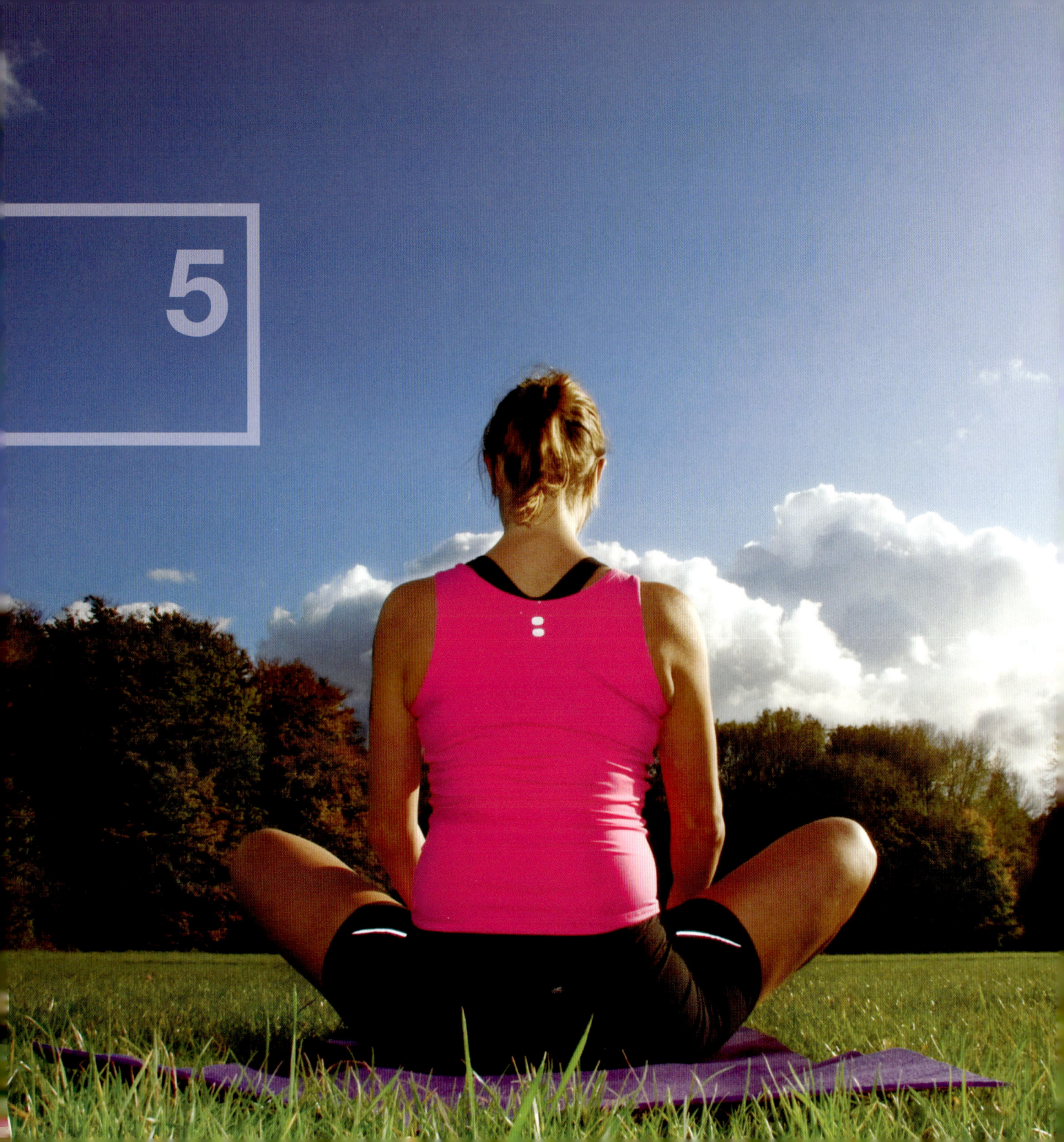

5

Exercises to relax

The following 2 relaxation exercises will prepare you for the delivery. It will also make you feel nice and at ease.

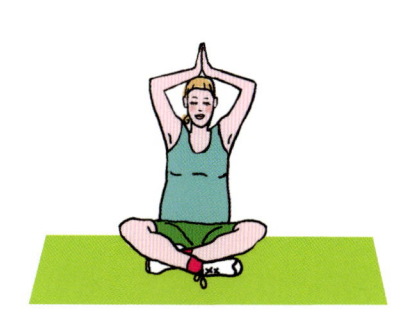

Cross legged sit
1. Sit down in a comfortable position, with your legs crossed.
2. Push the palms of your hands against each other at chest height.
3. Close your eyes and breathe in deeply through your nose. Breathe out and at the same time move your arms above your head and then backwards as far as possible.
4. Breathe in deeply and when breathing out return your hands to chest height again slowly.

Repeat this exercise 3 times.

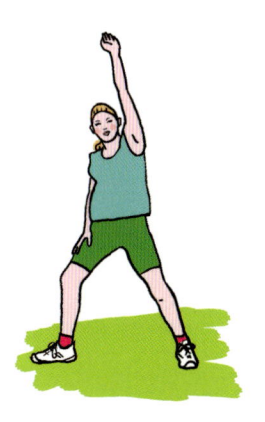

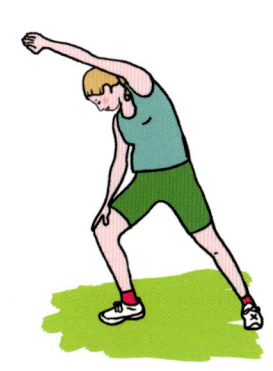

Stretched lunge
1. Take a big step forwards with your right leg while your left foot still points straight forward.
2. Go through your right knee and put the palm of your hand on your right inner thigh.
3. Breathe in deeply and at the same time move your stretched left arm upwards. Then slowly lower your arm again while breathing out.

Repeat this exercise 2 times with each side.

Ease - relax - settle down

MOM IN BALANCE

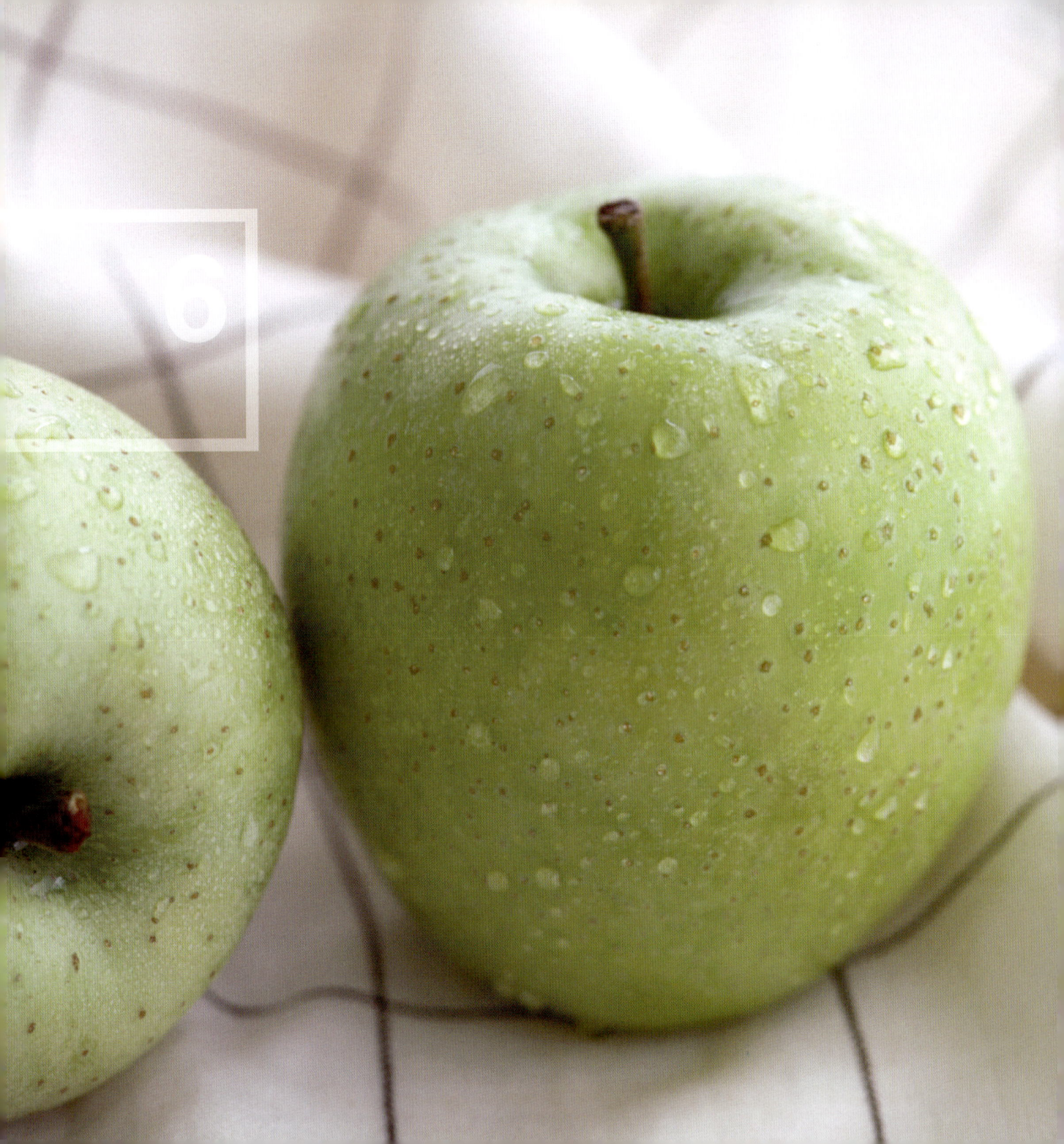

6

Healthy diet
during your pregnancy

In general a baby growing inside you does not even require a conscious effort. You don't have to think about your placenta growing: everything grows by itself in accordance with a great natural system. However, it sure is an exceptional effort, so it is good to help your hard working body optimize the growth of your baby. You can do that by watching what you eat, because what you eat has a direct impact on your baby.

Your baby receives all nutrients and oxygen via the umbilical cord. A healthy placenta is therefore very important. A healthy and balanced diet can deliver a major contribution here. Various studies show that a healthy diet during pregnancy offers lots of advantages for your baby. A balanced diet will of course also make sure you keep feeling healthy and fit.

MOM IN BALANCE

Nutrients

[Chapter 6]
Healthy nutrition

During your pregnancy, because of all the growing processes taking place inside you, the need for energy will increase. Many women already notice this quite soon, resulting in a bigger appetite. During the pregnancy you may feel you deserve something extra and every now and again you can give in, but if the need for more food strikes more regularly, at least try to take something healthy.

What you eat and drink is more important than how much. The slogan "If you are pregnant, you should eat and drink for two" has long been superseded. Now that you stay active during your pregnancy, you can use some extra energy, so you should eat a bit more. But still, not for two! Carbohydrates and fats supply the necessary energy in our diet, and proteins are used for the cell structure in our body. Below I will describe them all.

Carbohydrates
Carbohydrates provide the energy you need so much during your pregnancy for yourself as well as for the baby. They are stored in your muscles and liver as glycogen. During the first trimester your body is working hard and you use relatively more carbohydrates. This can mean you feel less energetic and more tired. When you are nearing the second trimester, your energy will return to higher levels. The following products make sure you get sufficient carbohydrates: whole wheat bread, unpolished rice, whole wheat products, legumes, fruit and vegetables.

Tips and facts about carbohydrates

1 During sports your muscles get their energy from the glycogen supplies. So when you exercise, it is important you eat carbohydrates for fast energy.

2 After you have been exercising it is advisable to restore your carbohydrate supplies within 2 hours because then it recovers more rapidly. This can be done by eating a filled wholemeal sandwich or 2 raisin buns and a banana or apple.

Fats
During your pregnancy good fats provide the necessary energy. They are also needed for the hormone production.

At the moment there is a lot going on about the essential fatty acids, or omega fatty acids. These essential fatty acids cannot be produced by our body, so we need to get them from our food. Our food contains a large amount of Omega 6, but Omega 3 you get mainly by eating fat fish.

Omega 3 fatty acids play an important role in the development of our brains and eyes and are therefore essential during your pregnancy. That is why health institutions advice to eat fish twice a week, of which at least one a fat fish, like mackerel, salmon, herring, tuna, sardines, sprat, eel and sea fruit.

Make sure you have fish on the menu twice a week!

Tips and facts on eating fish during pregnancy

1 Never eat vacuum packed fish like smoked salmon cold, but heat it first. This fish can be stored for quite a while and the risk increases that the Listeria bacteria gets a chance to reproduce. Heating kills those bacteria!

2 Salted herring can be eaten unheated. Herring is stored that short that bacteria hardly get a chance to reproduce.

3 Preferably do not eat any predatory fish like king mackerel, shark, sword fish, pike-perch and fresh tuna. They may be contaminated with heavy metals like mercury. Canned tuna is a good alternative.

4 Make sure you have lots of canned fish in the pantry: it's good food, with a long shelf life, and can quickly be tossed into various dishes. Use fish in your salad. Easy, good and healthy!

If fish is not your thing or you are a vegetarian, fish oil capsules with just Omega 3 are a good alternative. If you, being a vegetarian, do not wish to take fish oil either, then the best way to get those essential fatty acids in your body are a daily dose of linseed oil combined with algae oil, which are rich in Omega 3 fatty acids.

EXTRA CALORIES

During the first trimester you need about 135 kCal extra per day, which is e.g. a slice of wholemeal bread with butter and apple syrup.

During the second trimester you need 215 kCal more. Which is a filled slice of bread and a piece of fruit.

During the third trimester you need 620 kCal more, which is a hot meal e.g. 100 gr lean meat, 200 gr vegetables and a portion of potatoes or rice.

6

[Chapter 6]
Healthy nutrition

Proteins

During your pregnancy it is also very important that you get enough proteins. Proteins are necessary for the production of tissue cells, certain hormones and blood cells - essential for the growth of the placenta and your baby. As your pregnancy progresses the need for energy and proteins increases. During the third trimester the baby uses more proteins for the growth and development of the brain, so the need for proteins will be even larger. Products rich in proteins are cow milk (products), meat and meat products, fish, rice, grain products, potatoes, legumes and nuts.

Tips and facts about proteins

1 Another good thing about proteins: they fill well, so after a protein-rich meal you will not go hungry that quickly.
2 During your pregnancy you need to eat 300-450 ml milk (products), 1-2 slices of cheese, 100 gr meat and 1-2 slices of meat-product per day. If you can't handle that amount or don't like these suggestions, for whatever reason, do make sure you get sufficient proteins via other food.

Water

Water is the most important structural substance of our body. We consist of water for 55-60 per cent. It's in your cells but also in your blood and used as means of transport of nutrients and waste material in our blood stream. During your pregnancy it is important you drink enough. This will for instance support the constant creation of new tissue. Water is also necessary for a proper digestion. Each day we lose about 2.5 litres water via urination, bowel movement, sweating, tears and breathing. So compensation is essential to restore the water balance.

Tips to get enough fluids

1 Place a carafe with water in sight, as a reminder that you have to drink.
2 Try to drink a glass of water with each meal and each snack.
3 Make sure you take different kinds of fluids.
4 Start your day with a glass of freshly squeezed orange juice: nice and healthy, full of vitamins and fibres.
5 Drink fresh mint tea: easy to make and healthy.
6 Drink homemade ice tea: fresh fruit tea or herbal tea, sweetened with honey and served with ice cubes or grit.

MOM IN BALANCE

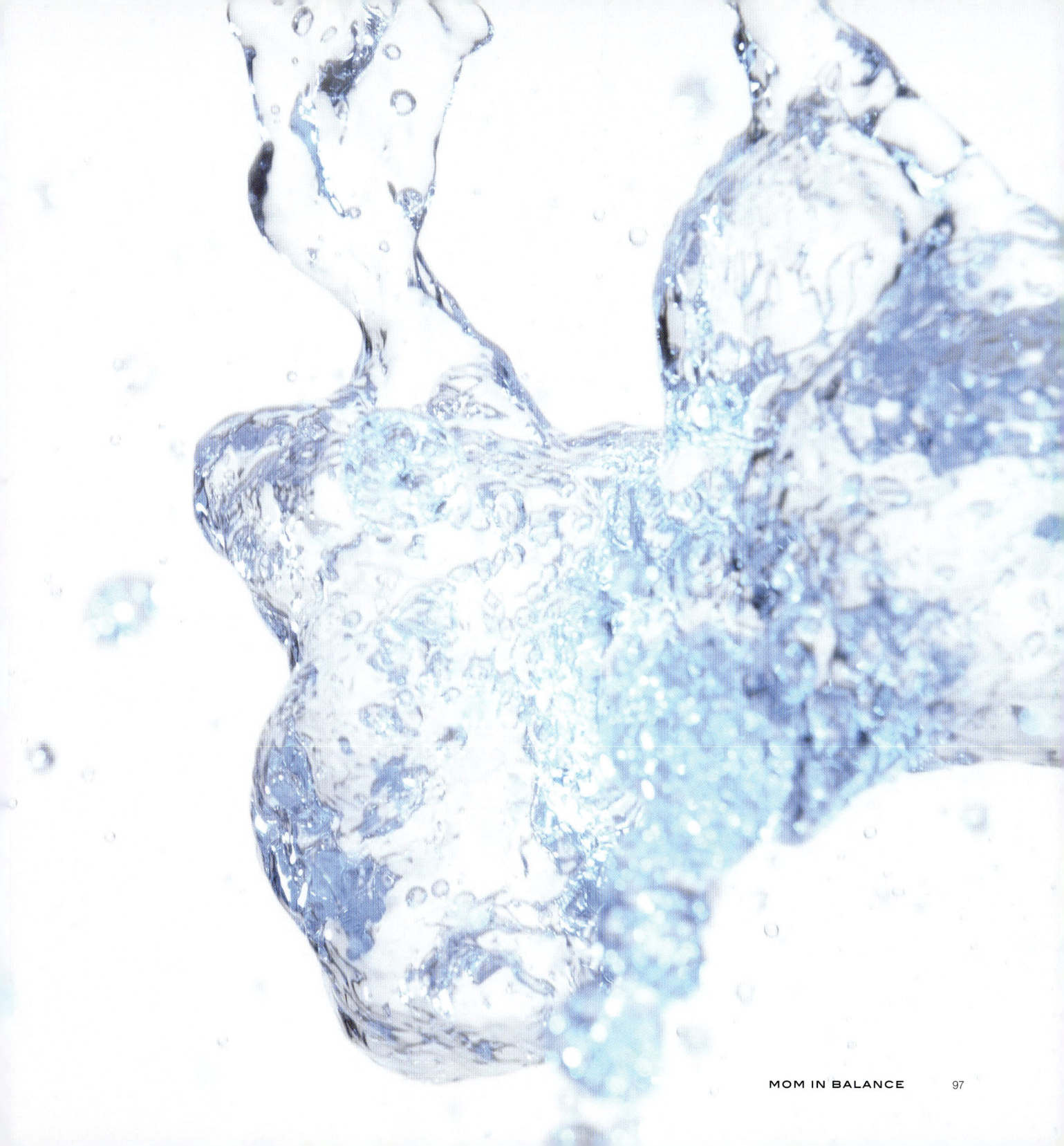

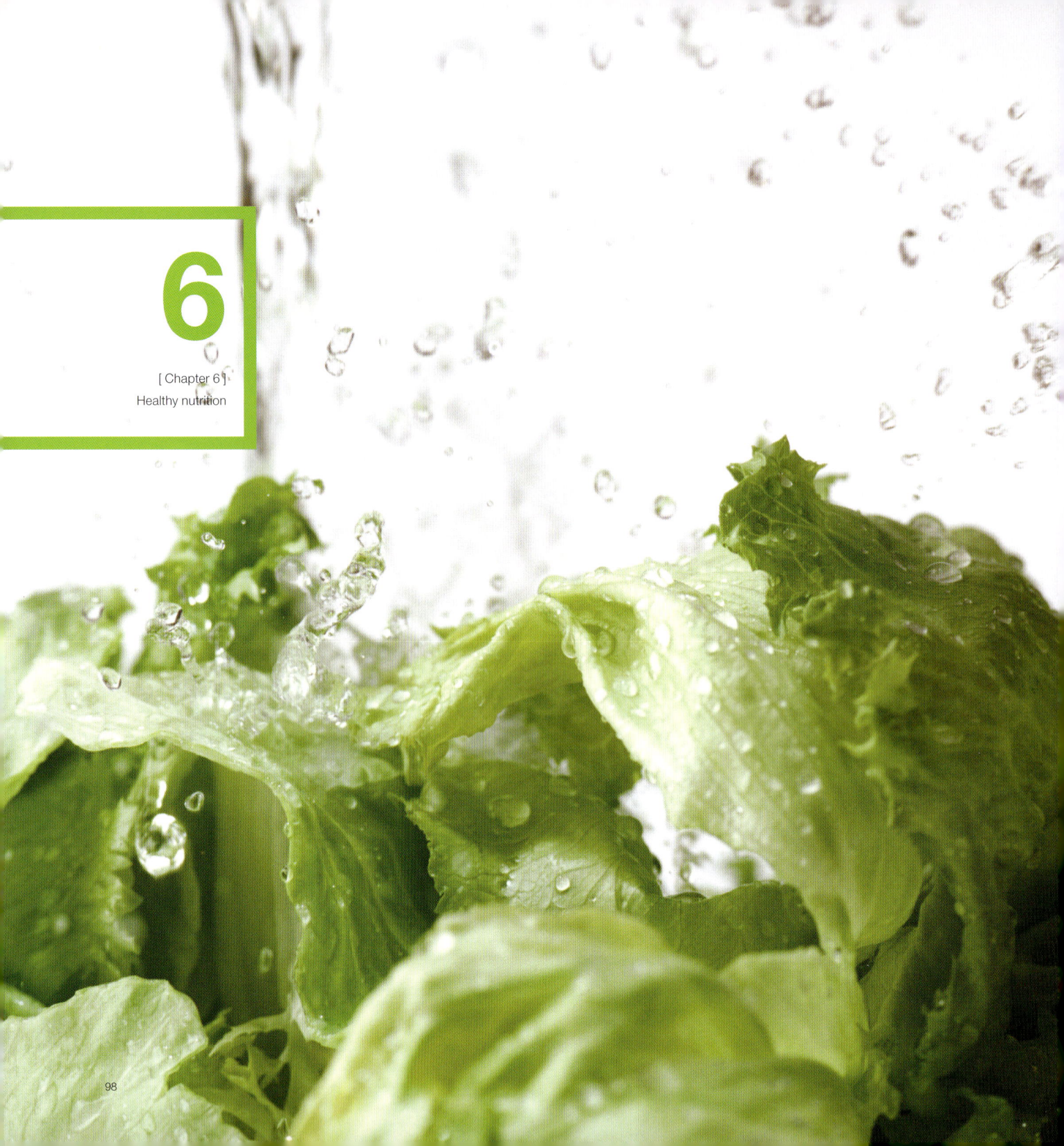

6

[Chapter 6]
Healthy nutrition

Vitamins and minerals

As a lot is being asked from your body right now, it is not so easy to get enough vegetables and fruit. But it is very important to take in sufficient vitamins and minerals. If you can't, taking multi vitamins is a good alternative. Do make sure you specifically take multi vitamins suited for the pregnant body.

Vitamin A
Vitamin A is necessary for bone- and cell growth and keeps your nails and hair in good shape. It also helps the functioning of your eyes. This vitamin can be found mainly in liver and for instance spinach, broccoli, milk, yoghurt and fat fish. During your pregnancy it is important not to get too much vitamin A as a high dose in your body may be poisonous. That's why you should take the special multivitamin for pregnant women, as there is no vitamin A in it. Avoid eating liver here.

Vitamin B1 and B6
Vitamin B1 and B6 are water soluble vitamins which are very important during the pregnancy. They release energy from your body and contribute to a healthy cell growth and healthy tissue. Vitamin B1 is important during the first and second trimester, when the baby uses more carbohydrates to grow. It also helps process your carbohydrates and to keep your muscles healthy. You can find Vitamin B1 mostly in fish, bread, potatoes, cooked vegetables, nuts and liver. Vitamin B6 can be found in meat, fish and milk.

Vitamin C
Vitamin C contributes to the cell structure, healing of wounds and the immune system. It also makes that iron will be absorbed from your red blood cells and is therefore very important during your pregnancy. You can find lots of Vitamin C in vegetables and fruit.

Vitamin D
Vitamin D is needed for the development of your bones and maintaining them. That is of course essential for your baby, but also for yourself. Health authorities recommend taking daily 10 mg extra Vitamin D in supplement form during pregnancy and breastfeeding. Vitamin D can be found for instance in butter products, fat fish and meat. The sun too makes that your body produces Vitamin D.

Vitamin E and K
Vitamin E and K are also essential during your pregnancy. Vitamin E prevents reduction of body tissue. You can find Vitamin E in sunflower oil, grain products and seeds. Vitamin K is necessary for a proper clotting of blood and contributes to healthy bones. This vitamin can be found in meat and green vegetables.

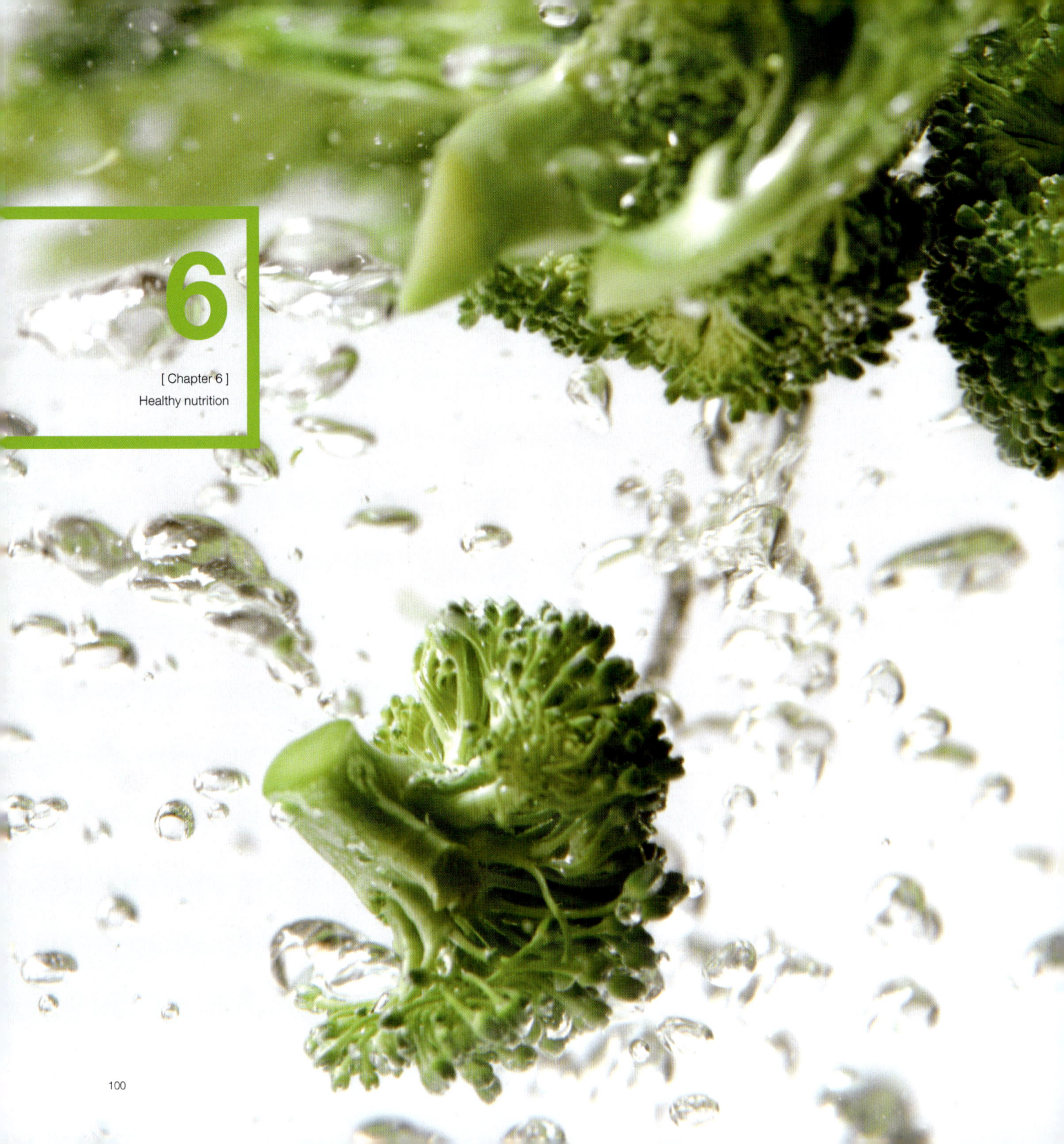

6

[Chapter 6]
Healthy nutrition

Vitamins and minerals

Folic acid
The intake of extra folic acid during pregnancy is very important. It helps the early development to go well. A deficiency is an important cause of birth defects like spina bifida and by taking extra folic acid you can reduce this chance by 60-70%

It is therefore recommended that from at least four weeks before conception until at least 10 weeks after the last day of the menstruation you should take in extra folic acid: 0.4 mg per day or by using a multi vitamin for pregnant women, which also contains the recommended quantity. You may use these multi vitamins during the total pregnancy.

Zinc
Zinc is a mineral that maintains your tissue. Next to that it helps your insulin activity, which is particularly important during the third trimester. It also contributes to a good immune system and the growth of the baby. Zinc can be found for instance in meat, yoghurt and cheese.

Calcium
During the pregnancy calcium helps the baby to grow strong bones. It is also very good for your own bones. Calcium also contributes to a healthy nerve system and heart and to healthy muscles. By doing sports you develop healthy bones too and it helps your body to retain the calcium. You will get sufficient calcium by eating and drinking milk products.

Vegetables and fruit
By eating vegetables and fruit you take in lots of vitamins and minerals. Fruit also contains lots of water.

Tips to eat more fruit
1 Plan that you get fresh fruit twice a week.
2 Eat fruit as a snack: easy, fresh and quick
3 Vary by putting fruit on your slice of bread: banana or strawberries or slices of pear and apple on a layer of cream cheese.
4 Make a fruit salad for lunch or dessert.
5 Dried fruit is a very healthy snack: it's full of fibres and vitamins and gives lots of energy.
6 Make fruit shakes or smoothies with different kinds of fruit.

Tips to eat more vegetables
1 Put slices of tomato, cucumber or pepper on a cheese or meat product sandwich: nice and fresh
2 If you have a busy job and vibrant family life, plan the meals for the whole week and do your groceries once or twice. You may even order it via internet and have it delivered: saves you the trip!
3 Make sure you always have a basis of vegetables and a variety of dressings in the fridge, so you can always make a healthy salad.
4 Healthy snacks: carrots, cherry tomatoes, cucumber, radishes, pieces of celery and pepper
5 Put enough vegetables into pasta, noodles or rice meals too. Or make a side dish e.g. green beans or a salad.

MOM IN BALANCE

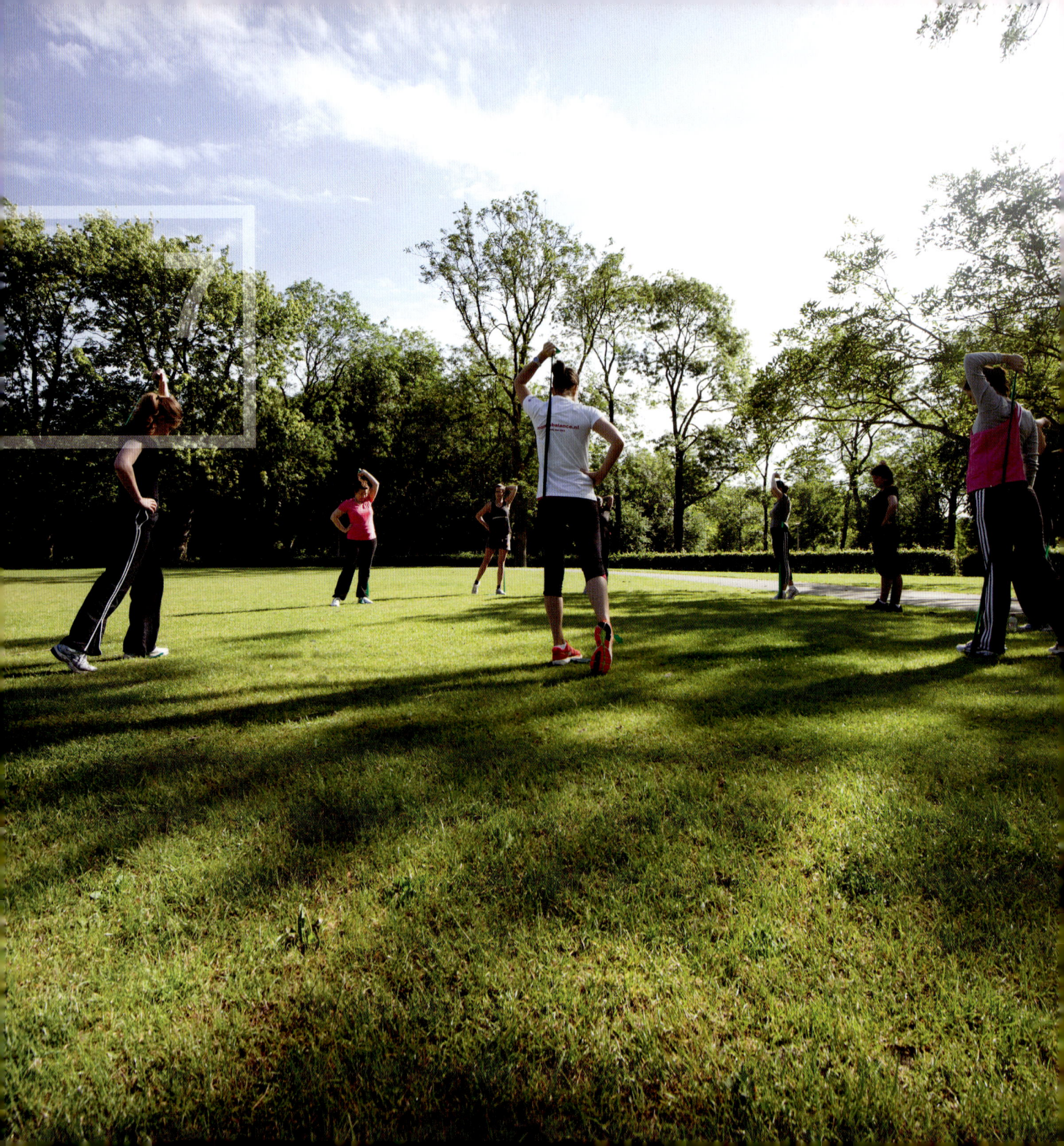

Recovery after delivery

Congratulations, you delivered a baby!

The first few days after the delivery can be quite hectic. Probably the first visitors are on your doorstep already to see the new baby and also the maternity nurse will be arriving soon to help and advise you during the first days. And of course all attention will be concentrated on the wonderful baby in your arms.

During the first weeks after the delivery it is important that next to taking care of your baby you have to take care of yourself too. The better you do, the faster the recovery will be and the more you can enjoy your baby.

The first six weeks after birth

7

[Chapter 7]
Recovery after delivery

The delivery is all behind you and now it's time for recovery. Especially if it's your first delivery you may feel all banged up. While your body is working hard to get back to normal again, there are also quite a few factors that do not really help: little to no sleep, blood loss, breasts filling up... And you've got your hands full with the new job: taking care of and feeding the baby! You may think there is not much time left to take care of yourself.

How will you find time for yourself in this busy schedule or to fit in any exercises? And should you already be doing any physical activity already?

To recover from your delivery it is advisable to take it easy during the first week and enjoy all the attention you get. In the past women were to take it very easy during the first six weeks, but now most experts agree that you can slowly build up your physical activities during the first six weeks.

For fanatic sports women this will sound like music to the ears but for most women it will mean an extra activity on their To Do list. From experience I know that during the first few weeks it will take time to get into action again and that it would be easier if you would postpone it for a while. But the advantages it offers, like a faster recovery, restoring your muscle strength as well as your flexibility and strong body, will make you want to get into action as soon as possible.

Build up your sports activities, take it easy

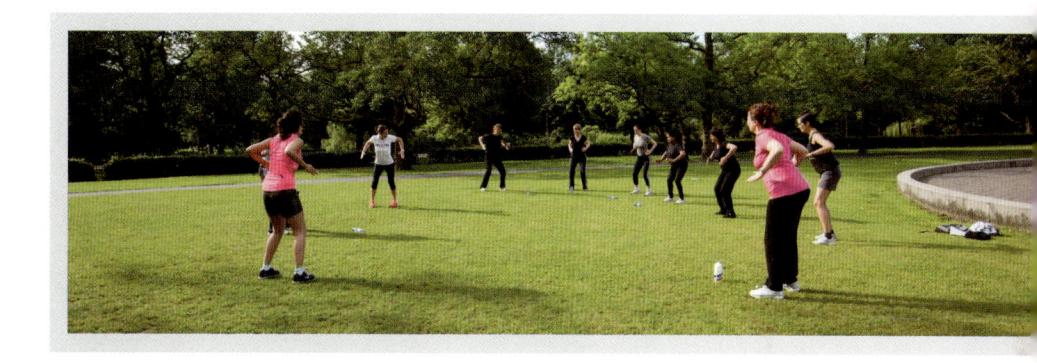

When you've had a C-section.
Recovering from a normal delivery is quite something already, so you can imagine that recovering from a C-section will cost even more energy. You've had a large abdominal operation, so you do need to give yourself extra time to recover from that. Not only in hospital, but also when you come home. Let yourself be spoilt by everyone around you. Here are a few tips to make your recovery as painless as possible.
- Accept all the help you get, especially during the first weeks when you really have to take it easy. So let everyone help with preparing meals, cleaning, changing the beds etc.
- If you are on pain medication, the doctor will advise you to better take them regularly, and not only when you're in pain. This way you will be without any pain on a constant basis, which contributes to your recovery.
- Take it very easy when you start building up your physical activities. In principle you can start walking and doing stretching exercises after two weeks, but do consult your doctor first to make sure. Watch out that you don't do too much immediately.

When you feel dizzy or sick, or if you feel the scar tissue pulling during the first weeks, do take it easy for a while.

MOM IN BALANCE

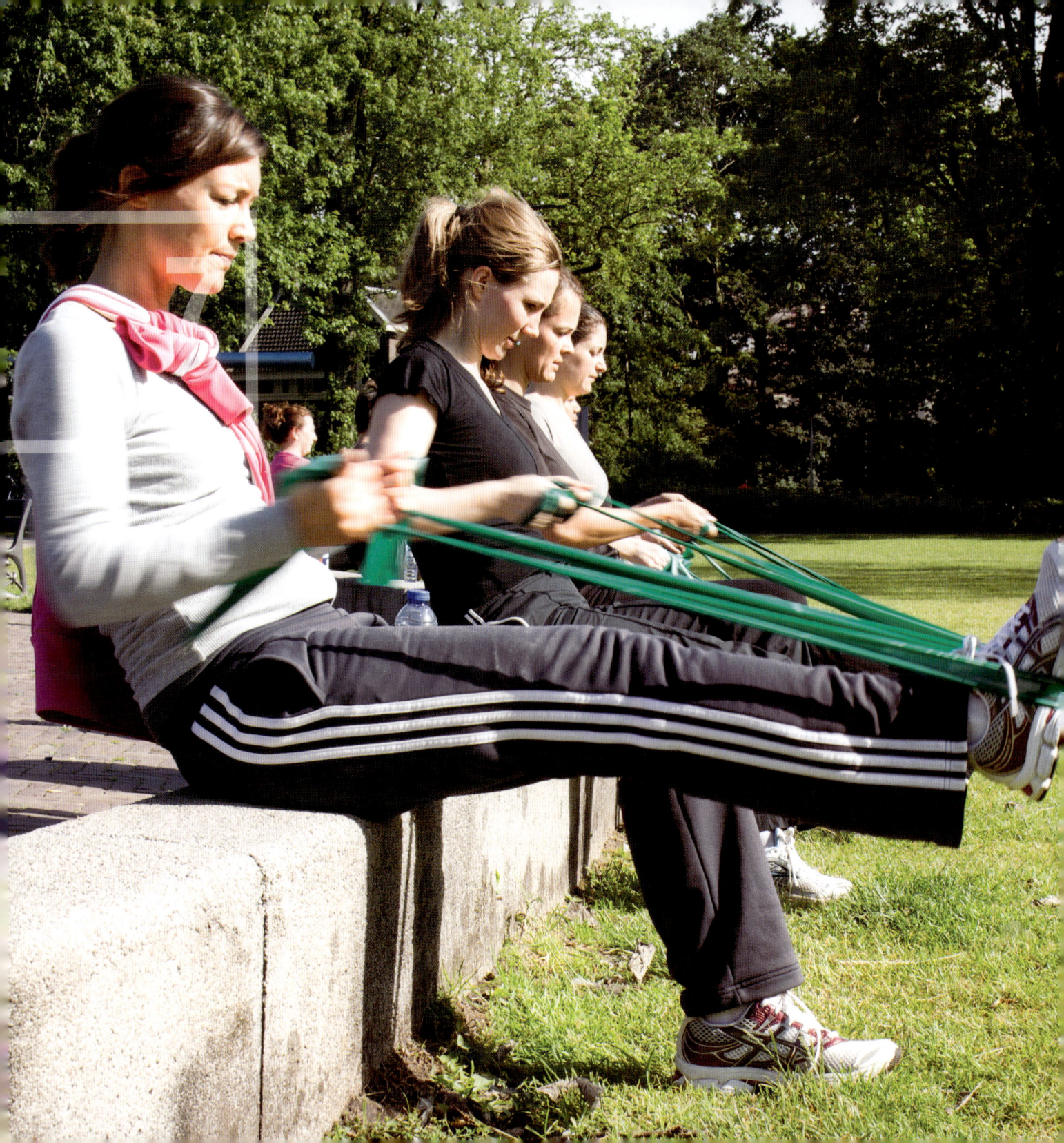

Your changing body

Sensitive breasts and breastfeeding

Immediately after the delivery your breasts will be put to work. When you want to breastfeed your baby, quite quickly after the delivery the maternity nurse, obstetrician or doctor will try to make the baby drink. This will help get the breastfeeding going.

The first weeks of nursing can be quite painful. The first few days of breastfeeding just hurt, especially with the first baby. Which is no surprise, because your baby will drink from your breasts at least 8 times a day in the beginning to get the necessary amount of nutrition and it's also searching for comfort and protection. The engorgement, which will start around the third day after the delivery, will force all the attention towards your breasts for a while.

If you breastfeed, it is quite normal that your breasts will stay sensitive during the first three months, but that pain from when your baby latches on will be much less after a week. There are a number of things you can do to ease the pain.

- Get advice from experts on what the best breastfeeding technique is.
- Put some of the milk after each breastfeed on your nipples. This natural way is still the best method to avoid nipple problems.
- Keep your nipples dry by exposing them to air in between feedings.
- Avoid using soap for your breasts, or rubbing them with a towel, this can lead to cracked nipples.
- If your breasts are quite engorged after the first few days breastfeeding, use cold compresses or cabbage leaves from the freezer to cool your breasts. Massage your breasts under the shower and avoid having your breasts almost explode. If the baby doesn't feel like drinking yet when your breasts are engorged, release the tension and pump out some of it.

When you breastfeed you will definitely have to wear a bra that fits well and gives maximum support. If you didn't need any extra support yet during the pregnancy, you probably will now. Your cup can be 1 or 2 sizes bigger than during your pregnancy. If your sports bra doesn't give sufficient support, I recommend wearing two sports bras on top of each other.

You will have to plan your exercises around your breastfeeding schedule. Especially in the beginning a tight schedule will not work yet, so try to be flexible. When you really start sporting again more frequently, try to breastfeed first or to pump milk out. Then your breasts will feel less heavy and next to that you will have the nicest milk for the baby. Because when you exercise you will have lactic acid being released into your muscles, which also makes your milk taste sour. After doing your workout that sour taste will slowly disappear again. That is why it's better to plan the end of your workout preferably one hour before giving your next feed.

Nutrition

When breastfeeding your body automatically loses lots of fluids, so if you do sports as well, it is essential that you keep on drinking, preferably water. Drink a glass of water each time you breastfeed and always keep a small bottle at hand during your exercises. The most important thing

Your changing body

[Chapter 7]
Recovery after delivery

for a woman during a breastfeeding period, is to drink more water, at least 1-2 litres a day on top of the recommended 1.5 litres a day.

You use about 500 calories a day extra when you're breastfeeding. And if you also started up your training again, you burn even more calories. Do make sure you eat healthy food, with extra attention for fish, vegetables and fruit.

If you are breastfeeding, you will easily lose the first kilos, but do not try to actively lose weight during this period. If you lose more than 500g a week, waste materials that were stored in your fat supply will be released into the mother milk, which is not good for the baby.

Vaginal pain
Even if you did not need stitches, you will still probably feel a bit sore below the first few days. Getting in and out of bed, sitting on a chair and going to the bathroom may still be painful. To ease the pain, here's a few tips:

- Hold a cold compress against the sore spot several times a day.
- Keep a bottle or jar with lukewarm water at hand in the bathroom, which can help reduce the burning sensation when you urinate.
- The first week make sure you stay close to and in your bed nice and comfortably, as this can speed up the recovery and you do not need to sit on a hard chair yet.

Usually the pain will be much less after a week, but it may stay rather sensitive for a while still. If you wish to go for a quiet walk after a week, let the distance depend on how comfortable it feels below then.

Blood loss after the delivery
The first 4 to 5 days after the delivery you may still lose quite a lot of blood every day, as if you are menstruating. You better use large sanitary pads for this. After the first week the blood will become darker and darker, which may continue lightly until about 8 weeks after the delivery. Doing sports with the large pads does feel less comfortable than with a tampon, but it is the safest choice the first weeks after the delivery. Keep an eye on the blood loss when you start exercising again. If it increases, you better take it easy for a few days then and start again later.

The abdominal muscles

Especially the first few days after the delivery you will notice that your abdominals will have to recover considerably. For each activity that you need to use your abs you will notice that they are still very weak. And if your abdominal muscles can't do the job, your dorsal muscles will have to do more. So do watch out when you lift something and use the strength of your legs. Especially when you are bathing the baby, it seems much easier to bend over, taking all the strength from your back. Try to stand up as straight as possible.

Unfortunately your abdominals will not recover by themselves. To make them stronger, you will have to get into action. Although you cannot do all the exercises for your abs yet during the first weeks, you can already start tightening them. Try to start this as soon as you can, maybe even already on the first day. The sooner, the better. Use the exercises given in this chapter.

Your weight after the delivery

The delivery already made you lose 5 to 6 kg. Unfortunately your belly will not disappear completely within a couple of days. There are a few reasons for that: your womb will still be bigger than normal for about 6 weeks. Also, your body is still retaining extra fluids after the delivery. About 2 weeks after the delivery your fluid balance will be back to normal. Wear comfortable clothing the first weeks after delivery, especially when you start exercising.

Of course you want your pre-pregnancy weight back as soon as possible. But during the first six weeks after your delivery it definitely is not a good idea to go on a diet, as your body is working hard to recover. Especially when you are breastfeeding, it is important to eat healthy. The continuous production of new milk costs a lot of energy.

Even without a diet your body will lose the extra kilos in a natural way, just don't eat too much. Doing sports can help you lose those kilos in a healthy way, it works best if you eat healthy too. When you are nursing you can lose weight particularly in the beginning. However, your body will retain a few extra kilos as long as you are breastfeeding.

Flexible joints

The relaxin hormone that made your joints flexible during your pregnancy, can remain active from 4 to 6 months after the delivery. This means that during the first months after the delivery you have to watch out for sudden and fast moves. If you really can't wait to play a game of tennis, you can do that, but do be careful. Keep in mind constantly that your body is still a bit less stable than before you were pregnant.

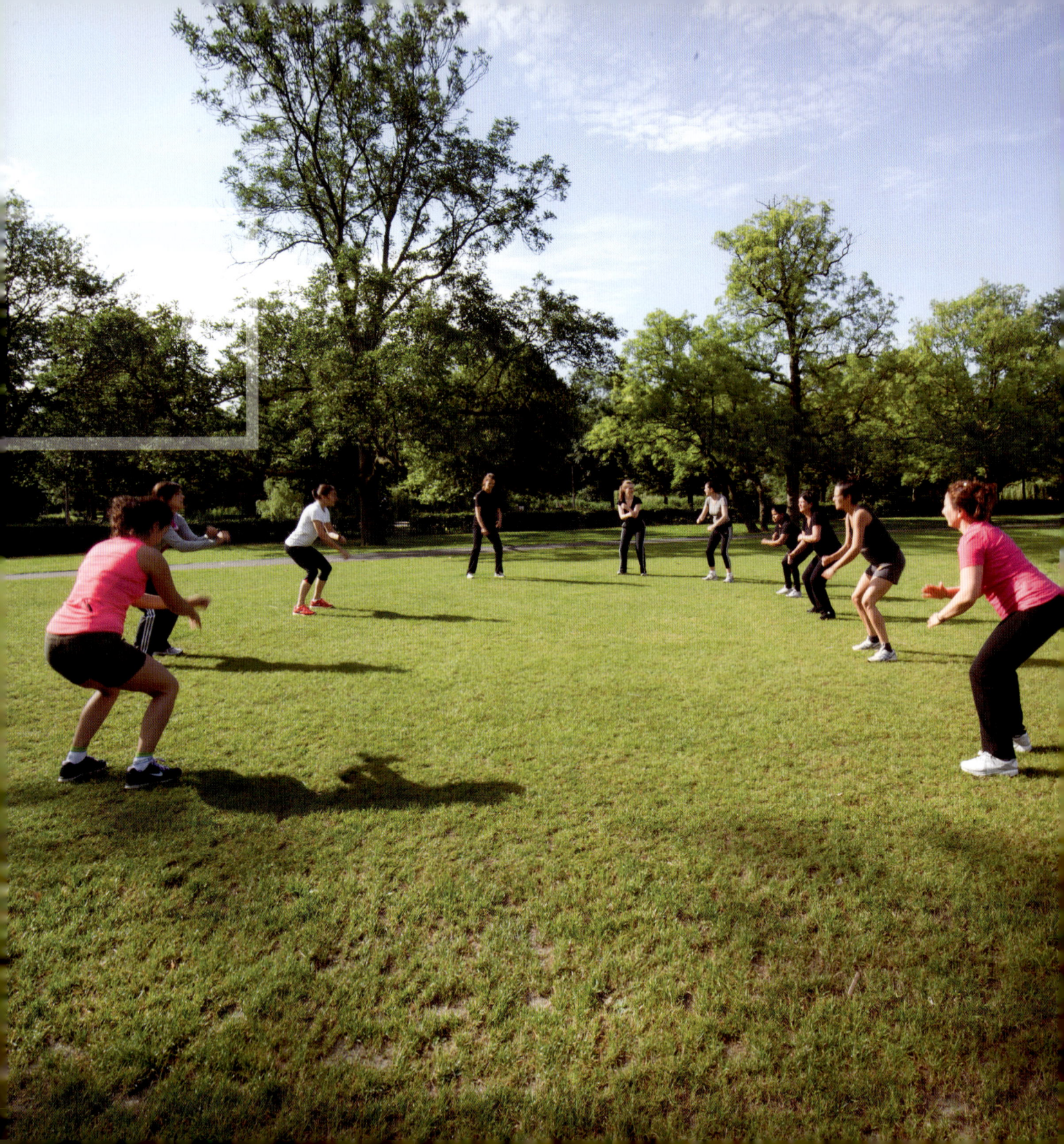

Exercise post birth

| Action 1 |
| Action 2 |
| Action 3 |

Particularly after a first delivery your new baby will be an extra challenge to get back into your sports routine. Everything is now about feeding -also at night- , caring, hugging and giving attention. And all this while working on your own recovery. So you sure can use some extra energy!

Getting back into action not only makes you lose weight and get stronger, it will also speed up your recovery. Start with tightening your pelvic floor muscles as soon as you can, even on the first day. This helps increase the blood supply and stimulates the recovery of stitches, if any. By strengthening your abs you will also provide a good support of your lower back.

The sooner you will slowly build up your exercising again, the better. I will advise you on how to build up your condition and how to make your body strong and flexible again with muscle strengthening and stretching exercises. The first six weeks will fly by because of all the hustle and bustle so have your action plan for the first weeks after the delivery to go by.

Writing down your action plan
Write down your action plan for the first six weeks after the delivery. Fill it in up here.

Recover, get stronger and build up

MOM IN BALANCE

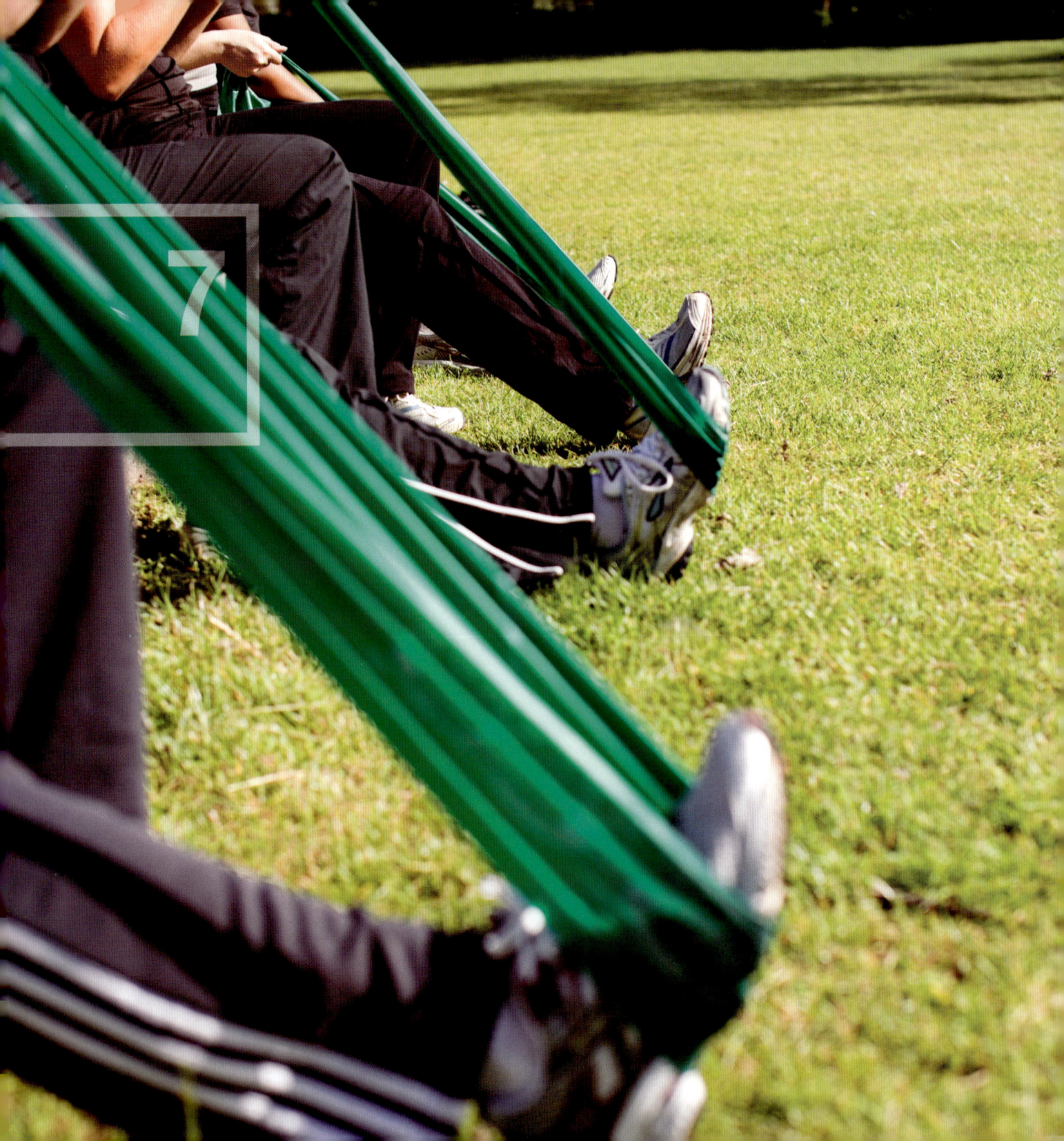

7

Cardio-fitness

Exercising will now be much easier since you don't have to carry the extra weight of a baby anymore. And if you managed to stay active up to the end of your pregnancy, you will notice that you have not lost much of your condition. Although you shouldn't expect to be able to run 10K after a few weeks already. Of course there are women who can do that, but on average this is not very realistic. Build up your training activities slowly again, and your condition will be back to the old level just like that.

The first weeks after the delivery will fly by. You're busy all day and don't know where time went. Next to that you will have to recover from all sorts of pains the first few weeks and you can be extra tired due to the broken nights. How do you pick up sporting again under these circumstances. First and foremost, stay flexible the first weeks and don't be too hard on yourself. Each activity is better than nothing.

The first 4 weeks
I recommend planning your first walk a week after the delivery. When you've had a C-section, consult your doctor first about when you can start your first activity again. Take the strawler and go for a 5 minute walk the first time. If this feels good, walk for 10 minutes the next time.

After this you can slowly build this up. Walk at a pace that you can still talk easily and make use of all the walking tips given in chapter 2.

Walking schedule
The first four weeks
Walk for 5 minutes at a quiet pace to warm up your muscles. Make each new walk 5 minutes longer until you've reached a 20 minute walk. Try to go for a walk at least 3 times a week and preferably each day when it is 4 weeks after the delivery.

4 to 6 weeks after the delivery
When the bleeding has stopped, you can make your walks a bit more intensive. To build up your condition more rapidly I recommend alternating a quiet pace with a fast pace. Start the first 5 minutes at a quiet pace, to warm up your muscles. Then walk faster for 1.5 minute, then slower again for 5 minutes. Alternate this with walking faster for 1.5 minute until you walked for 30 minutes. If it feels good, you can increase the faster pace time.

MOM IN BALANCE

Getting stronger

7

[Chapter 7]
Recovery after delivery

Especially the first few days after your delivery you may feel you don't have any strength left. But your muscles will not have lost that much of their power. E.g. your leg muscles are now in top condition as they have been carrying that extra weight during the last months, particularly when you have been doing exercises all the way till the delivery. Also your arms must be strong, and you can use that very well now, with taking care of and lifting the baby.

Your abdominal and pelvic floor muscles however, suffered the most during the pregnancy and delivery.

These muscles will not recover by itself, but need some effort from your side. The good thing is that you can start working on those muscles quite fast after the delivery.

On the side here you will find some exercises which you can do already in your bed and during the weeks after that.

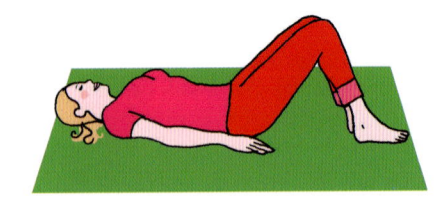

Abdominal breathing
A good exercise to start with to make your abdominal and pelvic floor muscles stronger.

1. Lie on your back with your knees pulled up.
2. Breathe in and out quietly from your belly.
3. When breathing in, relax your abdominal and pelvic floor muscles.
4. When breathing out, your belly will be flat again and the pelvic floor muscles will come up again.
5. Tighten your abs and pelvic floor muscles lightly during this exercise.

Repeat this exercise 6 times.

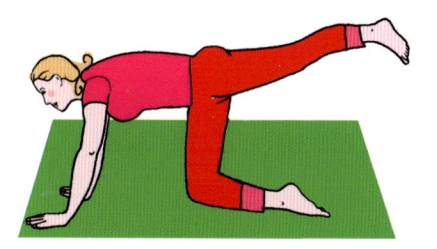

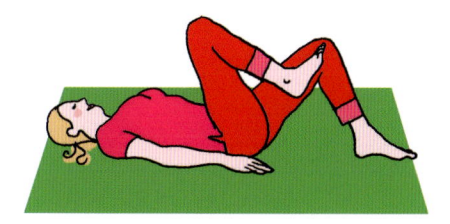

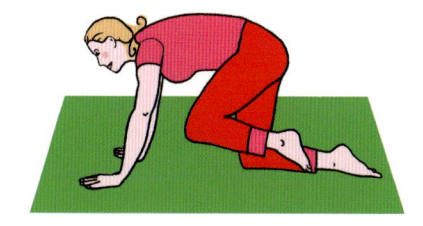

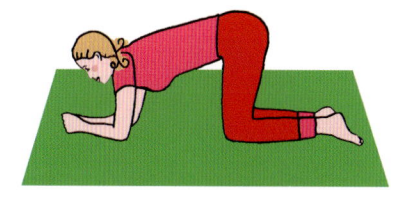

Leg bend

This exercise is good for the blood circulation in your legs and for strengthening your pelvic floor and abdominals.

1   Lie down on your back with your legs stretched and your arms alongside your body.
2   Bend your right leg to your chest and then stretch your leg forward again.

Repeat this exercise with both legs 8-10 times.

Backward kick

This exercise helps strengthen your upper legs and abdominal muscles.

1   Get down on your hands and knees and lightly tighten your abs.
2   Lift your right leg, bend your knee and move your knee towards your chest.
3   Stretch your leg again and lower your leg until your toes touch the ground.

Repeat the exercise 6-8 times with each leg.

Abdominal muscles

This is a good exercise for your abs to start with.

1   Get down on your hands and knees, then lean on your underarms.
2   Keep your back straight and tighten your abdominals, while pulling up your navel. Keep it tightened for 3 seconds, then relax your belly again.

Repeat this exercise 6-8 times.

MOM IN BALANCE

7

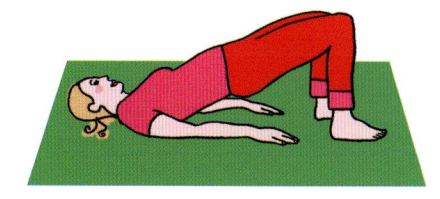

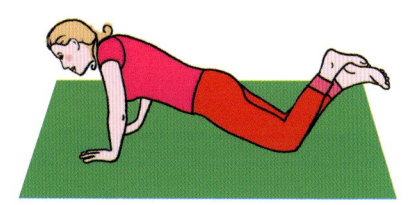

Bridge

This exercise is good to improve the stability of your body muscles again. You will also strengthen your pelvic stability.

1　Lie on your back and put your feet flat on the ground, slightly apart. Let your arms lie next to your body, stretched.
2　Pull in your belly button and tighten your abdominal muscles. Lift your pelvis. Your body now forms a straight line from shoulders to knees. Hold this position for 5 seconds.

Repeat this exercise 6 times.

Plank

The plank strengthens the inner oblique abdominal muscles.

1　Get down on your hands and knees and lean on your underarms.
2　Tighten your abdominals and make sure your head forms a line with your body. Don't arch your back or let your belly sag.
3　Hold this position for 5 seconds.

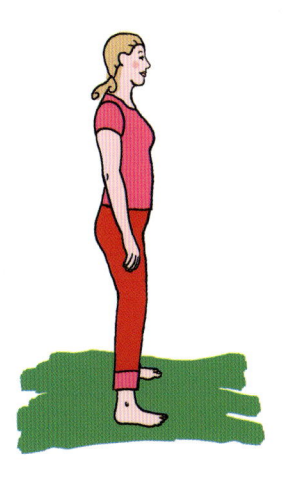

Repeat this exercise 3 times.

Pelvic floor muscles

To strengthen the pelvic floor muscles. Start as soon as possible after the delivery with the next exercise.

1　Stand up with your legs a little apart. Keep a relaxed posture.
2　Pull up your pelvic floor muscles and try to hold them tightened for 6-8 seconds.
3　Keep your glutes and belly relaxed while tightening your pelvic floor muscles.

Repeat this exercise 3 times a day with 10 repeats at the time.

MOM IN BALANCE

Flexible muscles

7

[Chapter 7]
Recovery after delivery

Next to the fact that it's very good to strengthen your muscles again, stretching your muscles will prevent all kinds of aches and pain. Stretching your belly, back, calves and hamstrings will soon make you feel great. With the following stretching exercises you can safely put all muscles back to work. Start slowly and hold each stretch for at least 10 seconds.

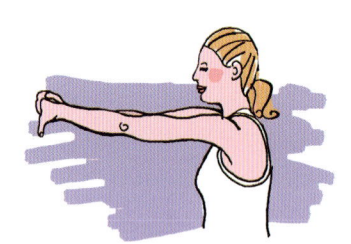

Upper back stretch

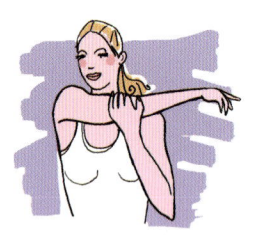

Shoulder stretch

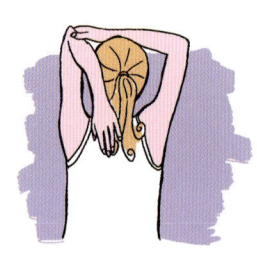

Triceps stretch

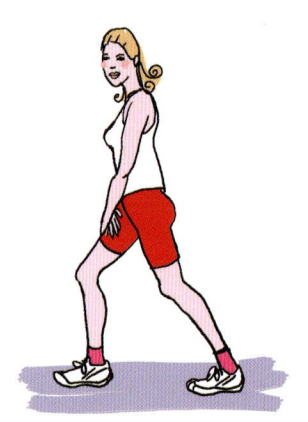

Calf stretch

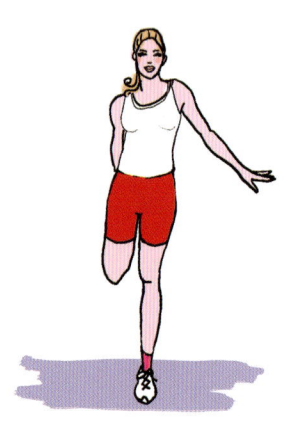

Upper leg stretch

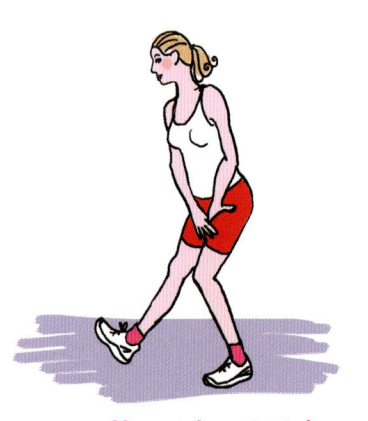

Hamstring stretch

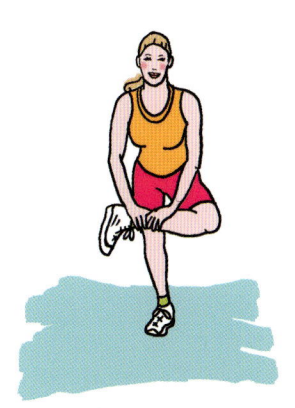

Gluteal muscle stretch

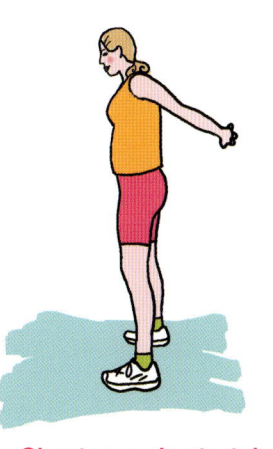

Chest-muscle stretch

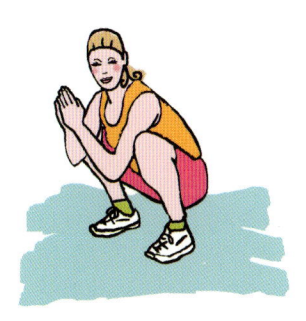

Lower back stretch

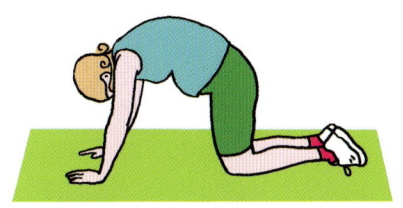

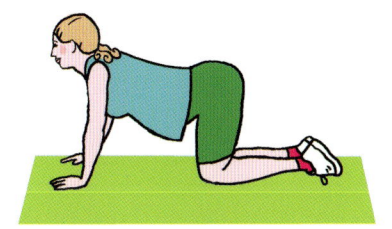

Cat stretch

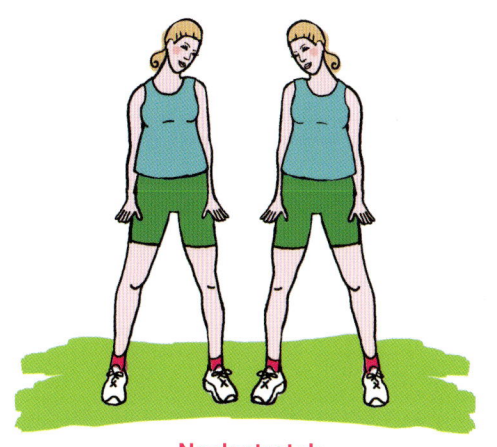

Neck stretch

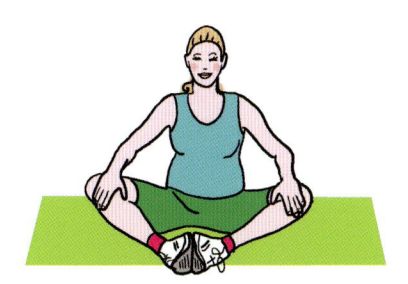

Thigh stretch

MOM IN BALANCE 119

Finally...

What a great achievement, being pregnant for 9 months and bringing your child into the world! Hopefully you perceived your pregnancy energetically and pleasantly and you managed to stay active and healthy all the way till the end.

Motherhood is something very special, each time again. You're busy taking care of and cuddling your baby and you will enjoy each step of his or her development.

Your family will get a totally new routine. And: the better you feel yourself, the more you can enjoy the first years of motherhood. So try to eat healthy and make some time to exercise. But make sure you take time to relax too. With a good condition and a relaxed and strong body you will get through those broken nights easier and be able to combine your family, job and all other things that are important to you, in an energetic way.

It is also important to let your body optimally recover between two pregnancies. The better you restore your condition, the healthier you will be for your next pregnancy, if any.

TIP

Check www.mominbalance.com for the Mom in Balance Back in Shape program in your neighbourhood. With these workouts in the open air you will build up your condition again with cardio-fitness. And with the muscle strengthening exercises and stretching you make your body strong and supple. You can start the program 6 weeks after the delivery and if you had a C-section, 8 weeks.

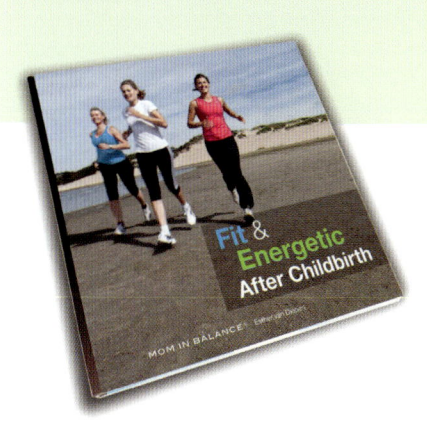

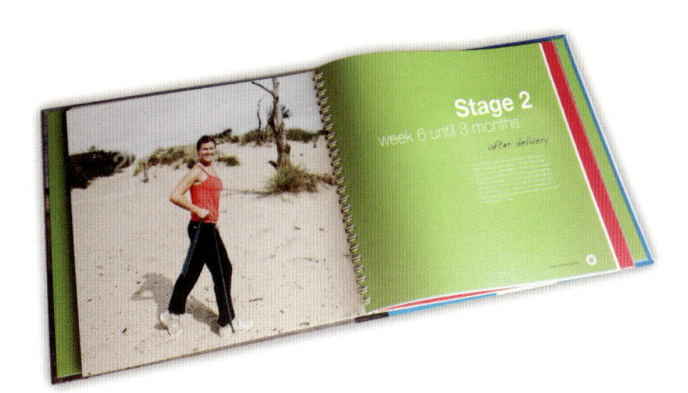

Check www.mominbalance.com

Journal

Make your notes here

In the nine month-fit journal you can write down what your action plan is going to be: for instance when you are going to run in the park or which stretching exercises you will be doing. But there is also room for records like how much your belly has grown or when you are going away with friends to be pampered for a day. You can also put up some pictures of your belly in here, or write down what strikes you or amazes you. In short: in this diary you will note everything you are going to do and what you're experiencing in these exciting times!

week 1, 2 and 3

mo

tu

we

th

fr

sa

su

*maybe you don't know yet
that you're pregnant*

week 4 and 5

mo

tu

we

th

fr

sa

su

Yes! I'm pregnant!

Date of pregnancy test:

week 6

mo

tu

we

th

fr

sa

su

first photo of your belly

week 7

mo

tu

we

th

fr

sa

su

week 8

mo

tu

we

th

fr

sa

su

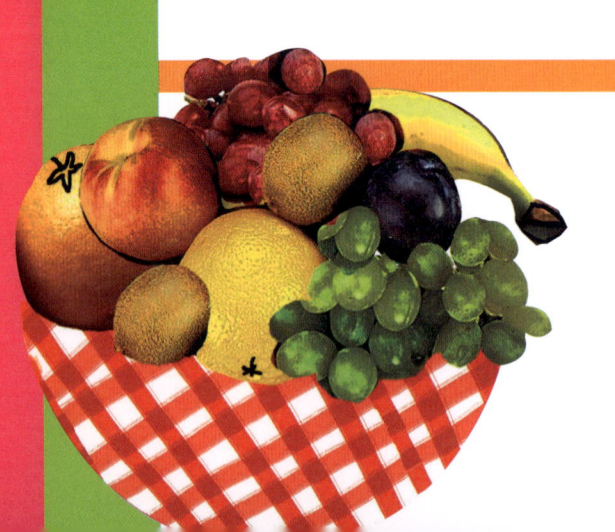

Make sure your fruit bowl is filled with lovely fresh fruit!

week 9

mo

tu

we

th

fr

sa

su

Hormones are racing through my body!

week 10

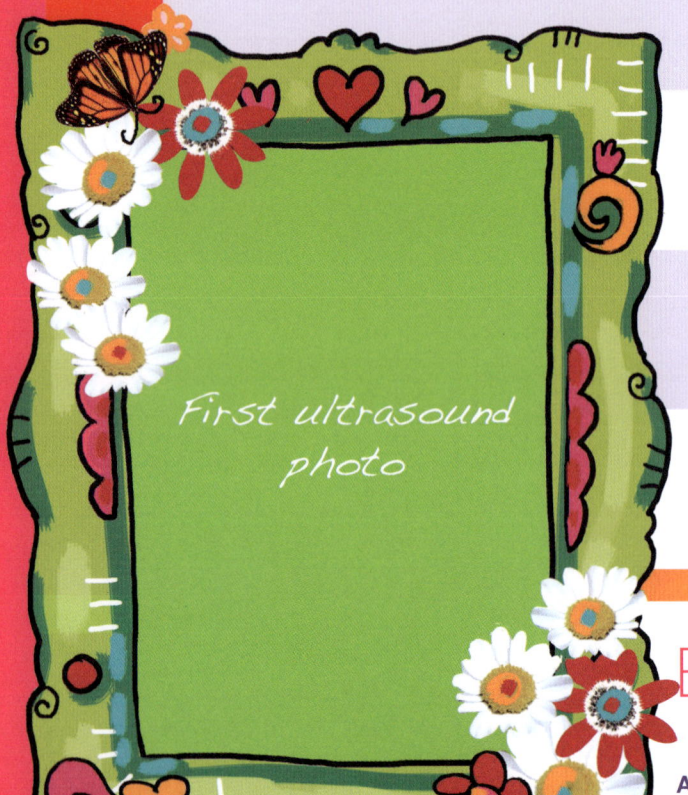

mo

tu

we

th

fr

sa

su

First ultrasound photo

Exciting, first ultrasound!

Appointment with doctor:

Baby due on:

week 11

mo

tu

we

th

fr

sa

su

I feel sick…

○ yes   ○ no   ○ a little

week 12

mo

tu

we

th

fr

sa

su

first trimester belly photo

week 13

mo

tu

we

th

fr

sa

su

To measure is to know

Belly size:

Weight:

week 14

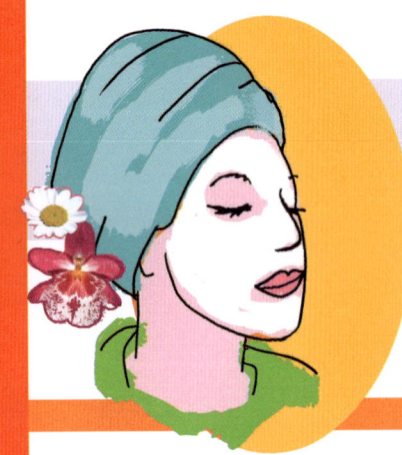

mo

tu

we

th

fr

sa

su

Tip: have a relaxing facial mask each week

week 15

mo

tu

we

th

fr

sa

su

The first trimester is over!

week 16

mo

tu

we

th

fr

sa

su

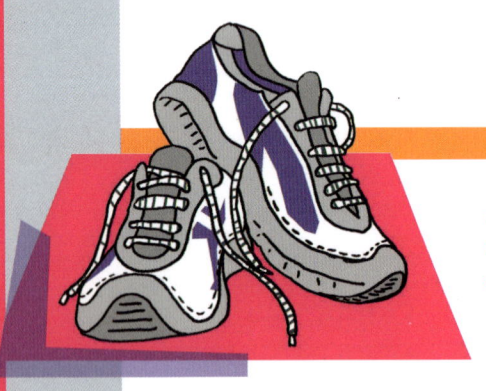

The better your sports gear, the sooner you feel like getting in action. If you wear properly supporting sneakers, your walk will be a breeze!

week 17

mo

tu

we

th

fr

sa

su

Go on!

week 18

mo

tu

we

th

fr

sa

su

You also have cool bathing suits for pregnant women

week 19

mo

tu

we

th

fr

sa

su

To measure is to know

Belly size:

Weight:

week 20

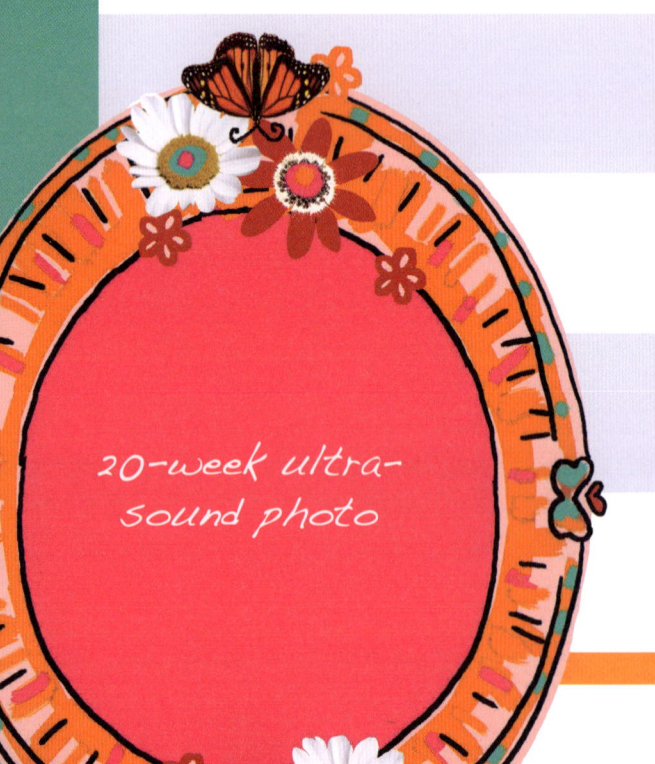

mo

tu

we

th

fr

sa

su

20-week ultrasound photo

The 20-week ultrasound, good luck!!

week 21

mo

tu

we

th

fr

sa

su

Do you want to know what it will be?
○ yes   ○ no

week 22

mo

tu

we

th

fr

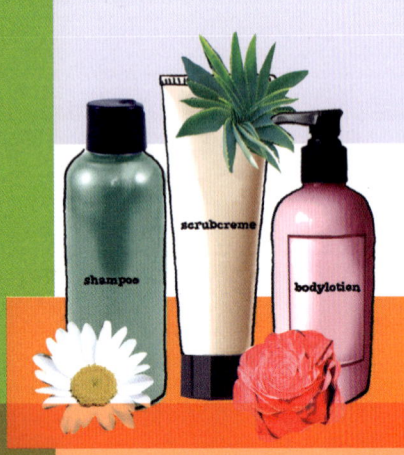

sa

su

Pamper-yourself-day

week 23

mo

tu

we

th

fr

sa

su

You're doing great,
keep up the good work!

week 24

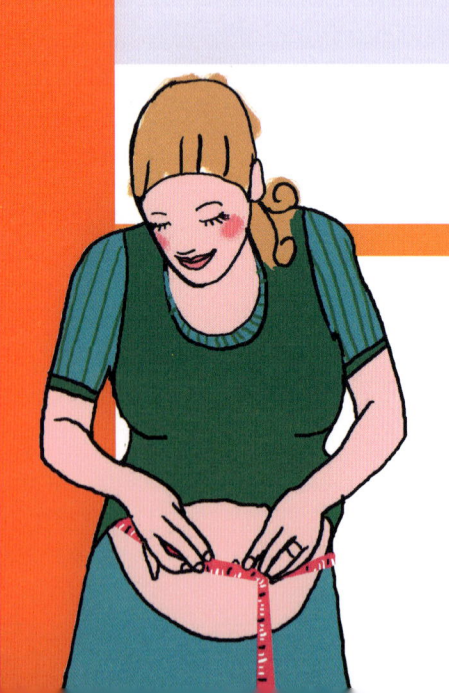

mo

tu

we

th

fr

sa

su

week 25

mo

tu

we

th

fr

sa

su

To measure is to know

Belly size:

Weight:

week 26

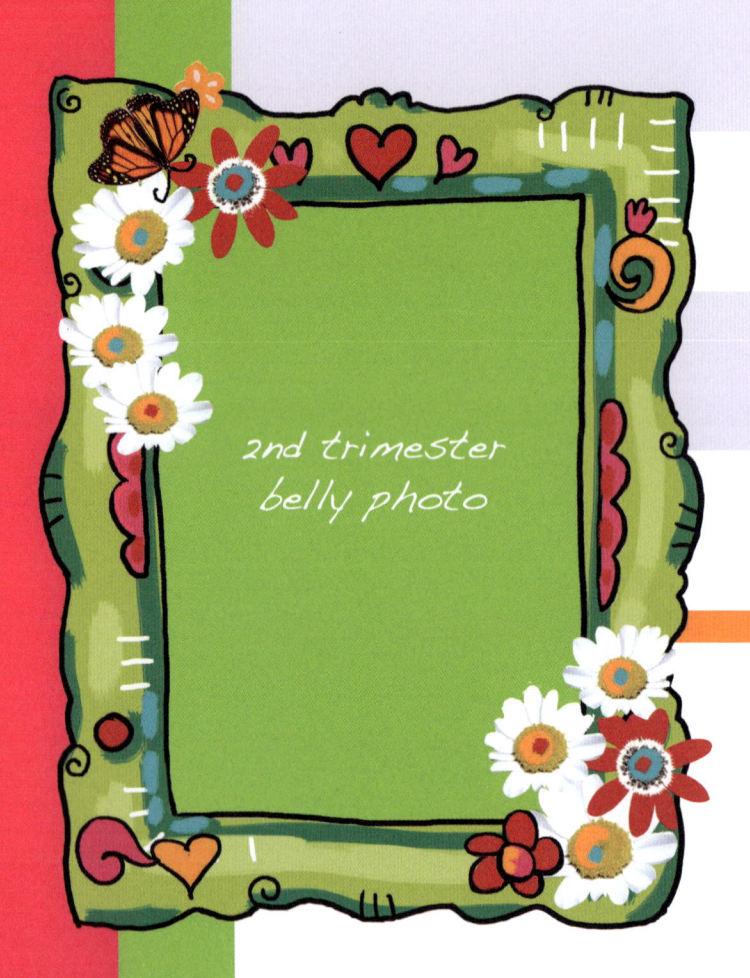

mo

tu

we

th

fr

sa

su

2nd trimester belly photo

week 27

mo

tu

we

th

fr

sa

su

The last trimester!

week 28

mo

tu

we

A healthy cruesli mix

th

Mild yoghurt
A tablespoon honey
3 tablespoon biological cruesli
Half an apple
Half of a banana
4 halves of walnut

fr

Pour the mild yoghurt into a large bowl and mix with the honey. Put the cruesli on top. Cut the apple and banana in small pieces and put them on top of the cruesli. Chop the walnuts in small pieces and sprinkle over the fruit.

sa

su

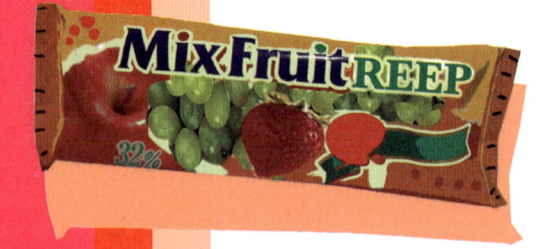

week 29

mo

tu

we

th

fr

sa

su

Am I going for a walk or swim too?

week 30

mo

tu

we

th

fr

sa

su

Take the Thera band with you when on a holiday!

week 31

mo

tu

we

th

fr

sa

su

Going for a nice walk in the park?

week 32

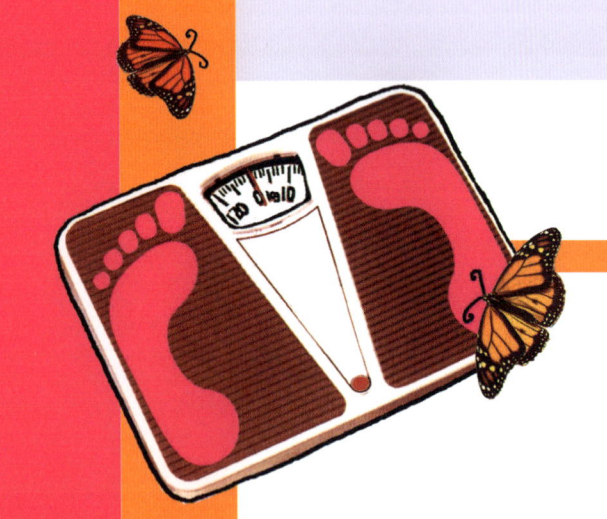

mo

tu

we

th

fr

sa

su

week 33

mo

tu

we

th

fr

sa

su

To measure is to know

Belly size:

Weight:

week 34

mo

tu

we

th

fr

sa

su

week 35

mo

tu

we

th

fr

sa

su

Some last shopping to do?

week 36

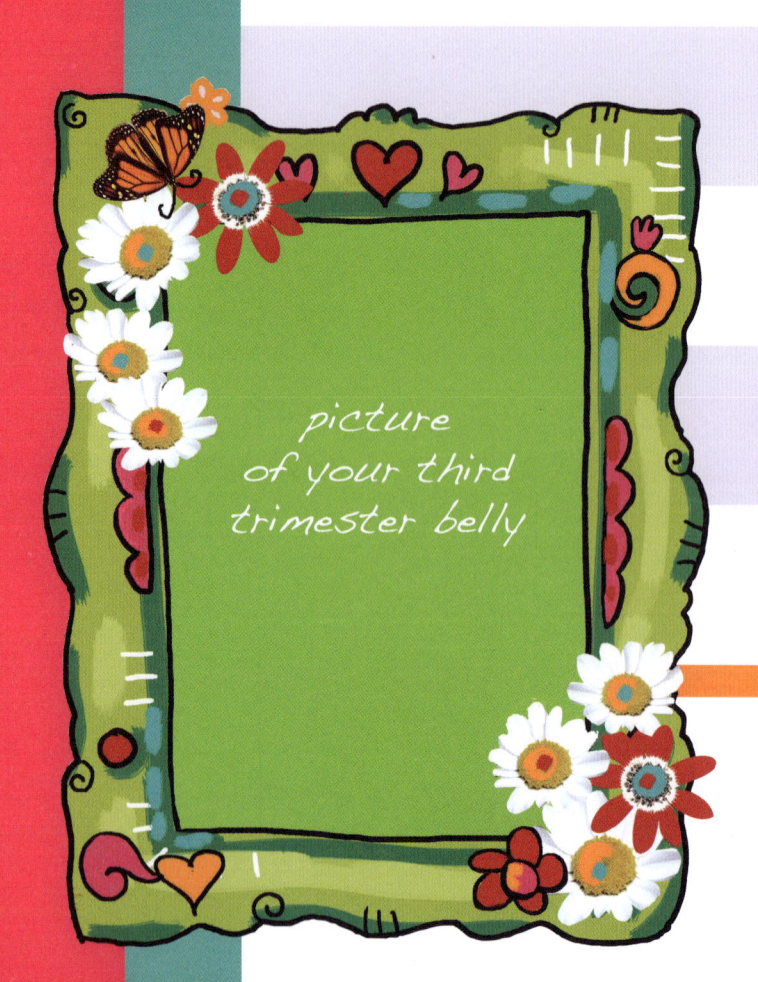

picture
of your third
trimester belly

mo

tu

we

th

fr

sa

su

week 37

mo

tu

we

th

fr

sa

su

week 38

mo

tu

we

th

fr

sa

su

Tired feet? Take a relaxing footbath.

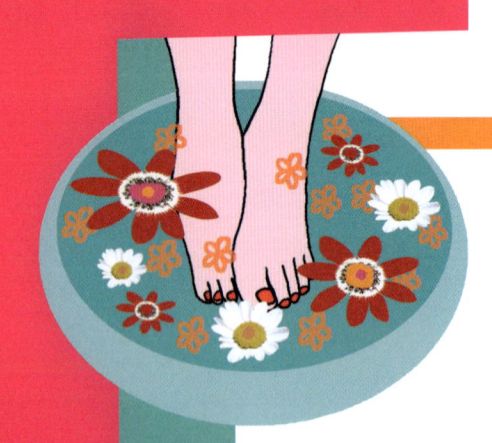

week 39

mo

tu

we

th

fr

sa

su

You're nearly there!

week 40

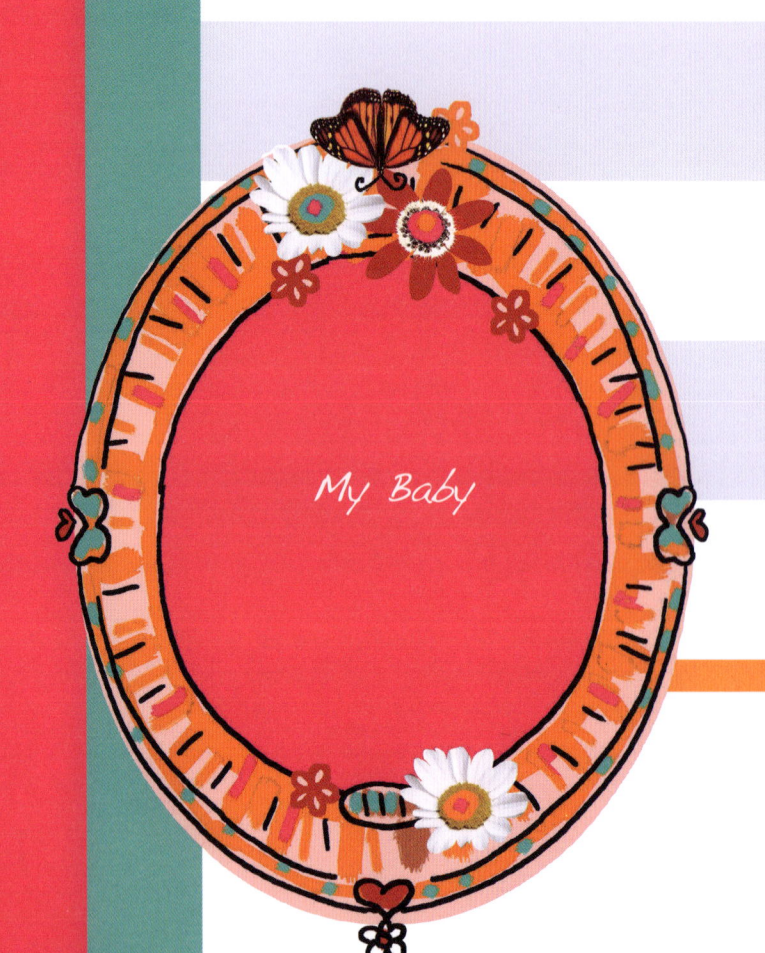

My Baby

mo

tu

we

th

fr

sa

su

week 41

mo

tu

we

th

fr

sa

su

Congratulations!

The delivery took:

week 42 and post-partum period

mo

tu

we

th

fr

sa

su

mo

tu

we

th

fr

sa

su

Overdue or…? Indulge yourself!

mom®
MOM IN BALANCE

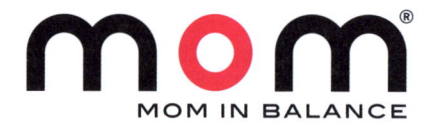

Mom in Balance
Work on your Active Lifestyle
www.mominbalance.com

Copyright © 2013, 2012, 2010
by Esther van Diepen

Design & layout
Alexandra Raddatz
www.logocompany.nl

Illustrations
Ingrid Robers
www.ingridrobers.nl

Editing
Louky Wagemans

Photography
Remco Liebregts
Esther Meisel, www.fotomeisel.nl
Marjory Haringa, www.marjoryharinga.com

Chapter Nutrition
Lilian Hentzen, nutritional expert
www.essentialbalance.nl

Medische input
Heleen van Kuyk, pelvis physiotherapist
Dr. Petra Bakker, gynacologist

Print
Publisher Services

ISBN 978-94-90510-01-5

Be careful and consult your doctor or midwife first before starting with the various programs from the book. Please stop immediately as soon as you experience pain or inconvenience and consult your doctor. This edition has been compiled using the necessary care. The author is not liable to damage as a consequence of possible inaccuracies and/or incomplete issues in this edition.

mom®

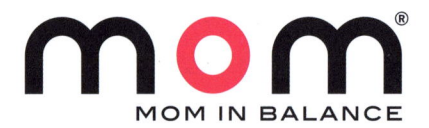

MOM IN BALANCE

Books used and inspiring websites

Baker C. Pregnancy and fitness,
Black Publishers 2006.

BBC News. Pregnancy exercise 'helps baby',
17 April 2009

Bermen Fortgang L. Living your best live,
LBF 2001

Boom-Binkhorst F.H. Mens en voeding,
HB 2002

Clapp J.F. Exercising through your pregnancy,
Addicus Books
2002

Clapp J.F., Rizk K.H. Effect of recreational
exercise on mid-trimester on mid-trimester
placental growth, American journal of
Obstetrics and Gynecology 1992
pagina 1518-1521

Costain L. En Graimes N. Gezond genieten
tijdens je zwangerschap, Spectrum 2008

Hendriks E. Lekker Gezond Zwanger, met meer
dan 60 recepten en tips. Caplan 2006

Jackson ea. The effect of maternal aerobic
exercise on human placental development,
1995 pagina 179-191

Keogh S. The complete workout log,
Axis Publishing Limited 2006

Meijer L. Hapsis-yoga voor zwangeren,
Akasha 1997

Moxley C. The busy mom's ultimate fitness
guide, Fitness InSight 2006

Nisbett R. Intelligence and How To Get It,
Norton & Co 2009

Paisley TS, Joy ea. Exercise during pregnancy:
A practical approach. Curr SportsMed 2003
pagina 325-330.

Rippe J.M. Your plan for a Balanced Life,
Thomas Nelson, Inc. 2008

Rock D. Personal Best, Simon & Schuster
Pty limited 2001

Swedan N. The Active Women's Health Fitness
Handbook, The Berkley Publishing Group 2003

Zwangerschap en Preconceptie 26 mei 2009
Den Haag, symposium over zwangerschap
en voeding.

www.fitpregnancy.com
www.gezondheidsraad.nl
www.voedingscentrum.nl

mom®
MOM IN BALANCE

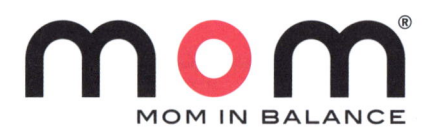

You can find more workout programs on the website or request a brochure:
Fit & Healthy pregnant, **Back in Shape** & **Mom in Shape**

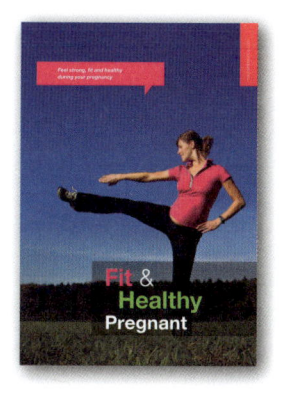

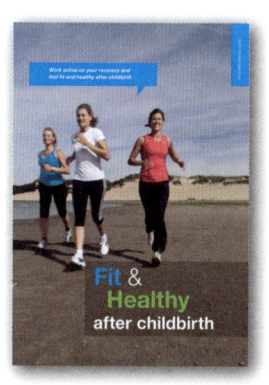

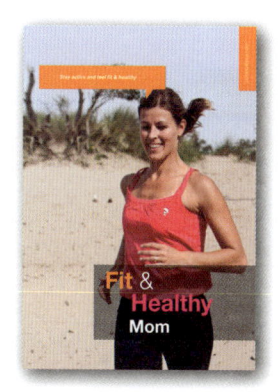